The Conscious Warrior

THE CONSCIOUS
WARRIOR

YOGA FOR FIREFIGHTERS & FIRST RESPONDERS

SHANNON MCQUAIDE

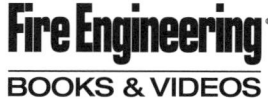

Fire Engineering
BOOKS & VIDEOS

Copyright © 2022 by
Fire Engineering Books & Videos
110 S. Hartford Ave., Suite 200
Tulsa, Oklahoma 74120 USA

800.752.9764
+1.918.831.9421
info@fireengineeringbooks.com
www.FireEngineeringBooks.com

Senior Vice President: Eric Schlett
Vice President: Amanda Champion
Operations Manager: Holly Fournier
Sales Manager: Joshua Neal
Managing Editor: Mark Haugh
Production Manager: Tony Quinn
Developmental Editor: Chris Barton
Cover Designer: Beth Rose
Book Designer: Robert Kern, TIPS Publishing Services, Carrboro, NC

Library of Congress Cataloging-in-Publication Data Available on Request

Printed in the United States of America

1 2 3 4 5   26 25 24 23 22

For my dad, Bill; my mom, Carolyn;
and all the women and men of the fire service
who have dedicated their lives to serving others.

Contents

Part IV

Part V

Part VI

Foreword

Everyone who witnessed the selfless, heroic, and courageous firefighters of September 11, 2001, was forever marked by their heroism and sacrifices. That's when I shifted my career to a clinical psychologist to serve firefighters and other first responders. Now, 18 years later, I'm more inspired than ever to help as many firefighters as possible strengthen their mental and physical health and wellness.

Every day, firefighters serve on the front lines of humanity's worst-case scenarios. They respond to terrorist attacks, mass shootings, motor vehicle accidents, suicides, murders, medical emergencies, and every other type of tragedy imaginable. In the course of their heroic work, firefighters are exposed to extraordinary levels of carcinogens, physical stress, and a degree of emotional trauma that most people wouldn't dare to imagine, let alone endure. And yet, firefighters endure it all, without end, and they make these sacrifices to keep our families and communities safe.

Fortunately, firefighters are exceptionally tough and resilient individuals. The average person on the street does not come close to possessing the courage, motivation, toughness, or outstanding capabilities required in order to function as a successful firefighter. On entering the fire service, the brave and heroic men and women who have dedicated their lives to serving others are portraits of extraordinary mental and physical health. They are the toughest of the tough, the strongest of the strong, and their courage is unparalleled.

Firefighters are at increased risk for a multitude of negative physical and mental health consequences, including depression, alcohol abuse, posttraumatic stress, suicidal thoughts, and suicide. Because the trauma of the job is foreseeable and the risks are known, these are predictable outcomes. Therefore, we must be relentlessly proactive in providing the most innovative and high-quality wellness tools, resources, and programs for firefighters. This is why the work of Shannon McQuaide is so important.

I met Shannon through our shared passion for strengthening the wellness of firefighters across the span of their lives. An expert in yoga and mindfulness, Shannon brings the most authentic passion and positive energy supporting firefighters you could ever hope to find. She is committed to conducting scientific research to support her work. I am thankful that she has written *The Conscious Warrior: Yoga for Firefighters and First Responders* and that you have decided to read it. Providing our nation's heroes with innovative wellness support is precisely what Shannon and FireFlex Yoga are committed to achieving on a large scale, to support and equip as many firefighters and other first responders as possible with tools and resources to improve their lives and strengthen their wellness.

Thank you to firefighters and other first responders for all you do. Thank you for your service and countless sacrifices. Your health and wellness are of the utmost importance, so please stay safe and well. Shannon will guide the way.

—Dr. David Black, founder, Cordico

Acknowledgments

This book happened because of my early champions who saw what yoga could offer fire-fighters and took a chance on me: former Chief Jim Frawley of Santa Cruz Fire Department was the first fire chief to say yes to FireFlex Yoga. David Dolson, division chief at the Roseville Fire Department and a yoga instructor (back when that was really suspect!), provided invaluable help with presentations and teacher training sessions. Chief Garret Contreras of Hayward Fire Department shared his dark night of the soul and how yoga practice helped him recover; he provided the content for my first talk at the California Fire Chief Association Conference. Chiefs Christian Tubbs of the Southern Marin Fire Protection District and Stan Maupin of Redwood City Department were also among the earlier adopters who bolstered my confidence and included yoga as an important element in their departments' overall wellness plans.

My sister Tracey Oliver, who was a firefighter for 14 years and is currently deputy fire marshal of Santa Clara County Fire Department, was not only my go-to person on anatomy and physiology but also was never afraid to say, "Shannon, that will make absolutely no sense to a firefighter." Dave Thomas, Travis Boelter, Mike Oliver, and Brad Morales-McGibben—firefighters who helped get the others on board at those early fire stations—gave terrific insights on how to make FireFlex Yoga work better and saved me from much eye rolling. And by the way, during my first pilot program, to help calm my nerves, Dave had all the mats laid out perfectly and had taped pictures of a couple of yoga deities in charge of removing obstacles to Truck 9!

I had a number of brilliant teachers who were important in my development as a yoga instructor. From Mark Stephens, Jill Miller, Sarah Power, Erika Abrahamian, Mariana Caplan, and April Underwood, I learned the foundations of my practice and found my voice. David Emerson was hugely influential in helping me refine how to teach for first responders. My focus on interoceptive yoga stems from him.

Thanks is due my friend Kathleen Ellis, who was a skillful coach and kept me optimistic and on track. And many thanks to Rachel Edelson, Charlie Harrison, Carol Day, and Renee Allen, who all read parts of this and kept me sane. The team at Fire Engineering Books & Videos was incredible; a special thanks is owed to Chris Barton, who was a champion for this work and is passionate about seeing more options to support firefighter fitness, and to Diane Rothschild, who pioneered a yoga column for firefighters and a yoga workshop at Fire Districts Instructors Conference.

I am so grateful for my sister Kristen and my brother John. Many years ago, I traveled to India and fell in love with yoga and meditation way before many of our family members were ready. However, they have always seen and appreciated me, supported me, and pushed me forward.

Finally, I want to thank my husband, Tom, who has supported me unconditionally and respected the work I've been doing for first responders since the beginning. His contribution cannot be overstated.

Introduction

Once a year, Menlo Park Fire Protection District in Northern California brings in a motivational speaker to present new ideas on operations and leadership in the fire service. The 2019 speaker was Jason Brezler, founder and president of Leadership Under Fire and an FDNY special operations firefighter in Rescue Company 2 in Brooklyn, NY. Brezler is also a decorated U.S. Marine who led several deployments in Iraq and Afghanistan. I was invited to this presentation because Brezler credits yoga and mindfulness as being important tools for creating a calm mind that can make critical decisions when it counts.

Looking around the packed room, I saw firefighters of all ranks. The conversations went from highly technical to humorous to devastating as everyone grappled with the challenges facing today's fire service: more destructive fires, skyrocketing medical emergency calls, an opioid epidemic, and strained budgets. Above all, there was recognition of a level of uncertainty and complexity of problems that can't be fixed, including the rise of the coronavirus pandemic.

In ensuring readiness for the "all-risk" demands of today's fire service, Brezler presented a framework for readiness comprising five critical skills:

- Define reality
- Build a cohesive team for a competitive environment
- Prepare through understanding
- Training
- Conditioning, execution, reflection

Pretty much everyone in the room agreed that as things stand now, *reflection* is the weakest piece of this readiness framework. Then, Brezler asked which leadership traits were most desired. By a wide margin, the top two traits were *maintaining calm* and *grace under pressure*. I was touched when at a number of strategic spots when he was talking about these traits, Brezler stopped and pointed to where I was sitting and commented, "You don't know how lucky you are to have yoga."

Why was Brezler talking about yoga in a presentation on operational readiness in the fire service? In a word, stress. He explained that once you learn how your body reacts to stress, then you can use tools found in yoga to self-regulate and better respond to stress, empowering firefighters with self-regulation tools to stay grounded and continue aligning their actions with their values.

Brezler and others in the military and first responder worlds are talking about expanding the concept of leadership from the *traditional warrior* code. In this culture, expressing emotions was once considered weak and feeling stressed out much of the time was just part of the job. The goal is to shift this to a more balanced, healthy, and, in the long run, effective model for not only surviving but also thriving in dangerous and demanding professions.

Interoceptive yoga, which is the foundation of the FireFlex Yoga program I bring into firehouses, is focused on building the physical and mental resilience necessary to handle high levels of stress and manage life's crises with equanimity. After several years of conducting classes across the U.S. and Canada, I continue to see how the skills that are practiced on the yoga mat—resilience, positive mindset, self-regulation, and self-awareness—are also essential components in good decision-making. Learning from our mistakes and being willing to grow and develop over time are essential leadership skills and support the *conscious warrior* ethos, a central theme of this book.

What's My Story?

How did an educator, entrepreneur, and a rebellious 20-something who ran off to India and found yoga and meditation ended up sitting in that conference room? The story starts with me growing up in a fire family in Northern California.

Growing up in a fire family

For me, it was a mixed bag to grow up in a fire family. I idolized my father and liked nothing more than hanging out with him in the backyard on summer nights as he barbecued chicken and told stories (fig. I–1). There were also years of watching my dad, a firefighter for more than 30 years, struggle with the impacts of a job that included injuries like a herniated cervical disc and tears to both rotator cuffs requiring surgery.

My father loved being a firefighter and said fondly, "You never knew what was going to happen at the firehouse." He totally believed that this job was for people who did not

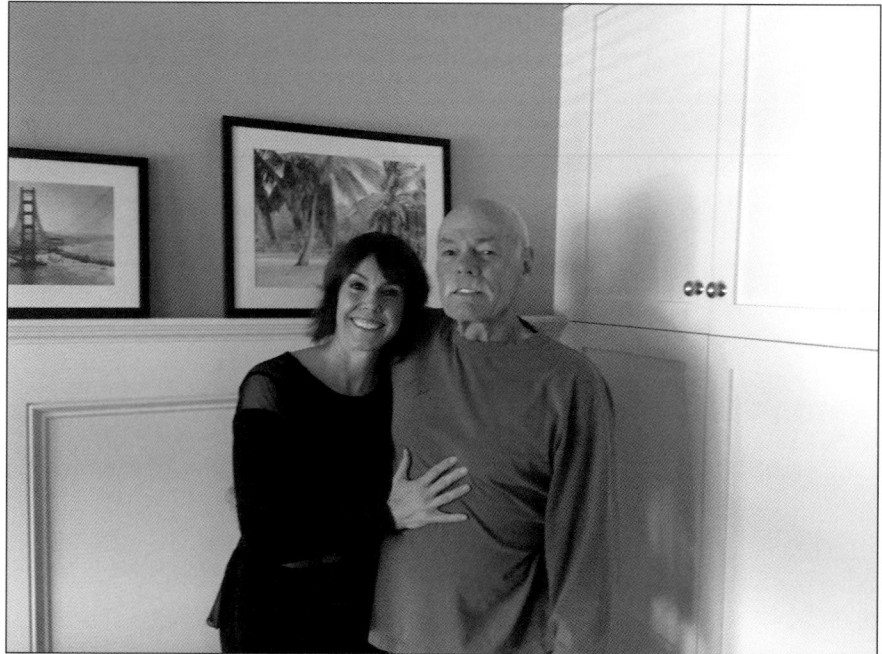

Figure I–1.
Me and my dad, retired firefighter Bill McQuaide

whine and went out there and did their duty. What mattered was devotion to the job, having fun, and having the back of your fellow firefighters.

Families of firefighters must deal with the consequences of living with first responders who are unaware, are unwilling, or lack the skills to talk about and process both the extremes of the job and the rigor of the daily grind. First responders deal with every kind of situation and emotion: violence, anger, death, neglect, mindless suffering. Repeated call after call, day after day, this can become like a corrosive drip, drip, drip of stress that can affect body and soul. Not having the tools to talk in a constructive way about personal pain, guilt, shame, and vulnerability can result in explosive anger, drinking to excess or abusing drugs, emotional distance, infidelity, and depression—outcomes from trying to live up to the expectations of the warrior culture within the fire service.

On reflection, I suspect that my dad was mostly unaware that the work he was doing would have any emotional or psychological impact. He worked with the same group of firefighters for years, including Terry Ryan, Morris Pisciotta, George Mattucci, and Ed Solano. They went on the same calls together, came back to the firehouse together, shared some dark humor, and were ready for the next call when it came in. Getting the job done, not talking about it, trying to compartmentalize—this was the normal behavior expected of firefighters of my dad's generation.

What affected me most as a kid was the lack of awareness that a psychological injury can be as debilitating as a herniated disc. My parents divorced when I was six years old, leaving me angry and afraid. There were no adults around (even when there were plenty of people more than 18 years old) to tell us—and me especially as the oldest—that this wasn't our fault, that it was okay not to be ashamed for feeling angry or helpless, and that we didn't have to pretend everything was fine.

So how did I deal? I became an alpha female. I emulated what I saw my father doing, sucking it up and being tough, not letting on that I cried myself to sleep many nights. I relished being aggressive and pretended to be thick-skinned and in control. I led with my anger and had few tools to de-escalate my own rage. Ultimately, I became angry and combative. These ways of navigating life, however, were shortsighted and short-lived. By the time I hit my mid-20s, I was tired of carrying around the painful events of my past. I wanted to understand why life (and my life) had been so full of conflict, finger pointing, and pain.

I became a seeker. I traveled halfway across the globe to get away from my family patterning and find another way to live. I encountered yoga and meditation in India, a culture and mindset that was so different from the way I grew up that it opened up an exciting sense of possibility: Could I change? Could I lead my life differently from what I observed growing up?

Did the alpha female learn anything?

Reaching out for help, I used a combination of therapy, yoga, and mediation, which together saved my life. I learned that although it may feel natural to turn away from fear and discomfort, doing so is often fueled by an unwillingness to be honest about our pain and express vulnerability. But what was most transformative and inspired me years later to write this book is the understanding that positive change is possible when we take the difficult step of admitting we are not invincible; instead, we are humans who thrive in supportive communities where we feel accepted for who we are and trust that we can express our vulnerability as well our strengths.

Yoga is a tool

Think of yoga and meditation as tools to develop an open, growth-oriented mindset and to learn to feel less afraid of and more comfortable embracing our common humanity. Rather than living life on autopilot or according to dysfunctional or unhelpful family and cultural patterns, yoga and mindfulness allow us to choose: Who am I? What do I value? How do I align my behavior with my values? And essentially, who do I want to be, especially in times of great challenge?

I still consider myself a badass, but my definition has changed. Even my dad opened up his belief system a bit. Sadly, he died of chronic obstructive pulmonary disease (COPD) just as I was finishing this book, but during the writing of it, he was excited and wanted to help. When I asked him if anyone was doing yoga in the firehouse during his tenure, he exclaimed, "No way!" When I asked him what the likelihood was of getting firefighters to practice yoga now, he said 50%. This was higher than I had anticipated. Why? Because, in his opinion, firefighters are better informed today. Surprisingly, he confessed that he wished he had been introduced to yoga earlier in his life! In bringing yoga into the firehouse, I've found a way to bridge the gap between us: East meets West, traditional warrior culture meets conscious warrior culture.

But did I ever say it was easy?

The Pilot Program: Shannon Learns the Hard Way

I'm pulling up to Station 9 at the San Jose Fire Department (SJFD). It's March 2014 and I'm about to begin the pilot program of what will become FireFlex Yoga. Station 9 had been my dad's and his brother's station for years, and I see that the same sign—Animal House (which I heard was my uncle's doing). The words *animal house* are painted on the backboard of a basketball hoop which was installed outside between the two apparatus bay doors.

I'm exceedingly nervous because my dad always said there are two things firefighters hate: the way things are and change. On the pro side, I know the group will give me the benefit of the doubt because, even when he was retired, Bill McQuaide was known as a good man and a great firefighter (fig. I–2).

On the con side, I know that yoga in the fire station could be threatening to tradition. Had I attempted to bring yoga to SJFD ten, or even five, years earlier, the firefighters might have laughed me out of the station, regardless of who my father was. The timing of this opportunity cannot be understated.

To combat my fear during the pilot program, I did a number of things wrong. First, I fell back on my own teacher training and practice, which relied heavily on providing precise cues with lots of talking and explanations. Did I say this wasn't my wisest decision? This is what the first classes looked like: sitting on the floor, eyes closed in silence, followed by a 55-minute boot camp–style sequence and ending in a 5-minute *Savasana* (corpse pose), which means lying on your back and basically not moving. Spitting out orders on what to do, saying things like "Root down through the feet!" "Press the inner palm down and lift up out of the wrists." "Feel the sensation of energy running through your body and let your heart bloom forward!"

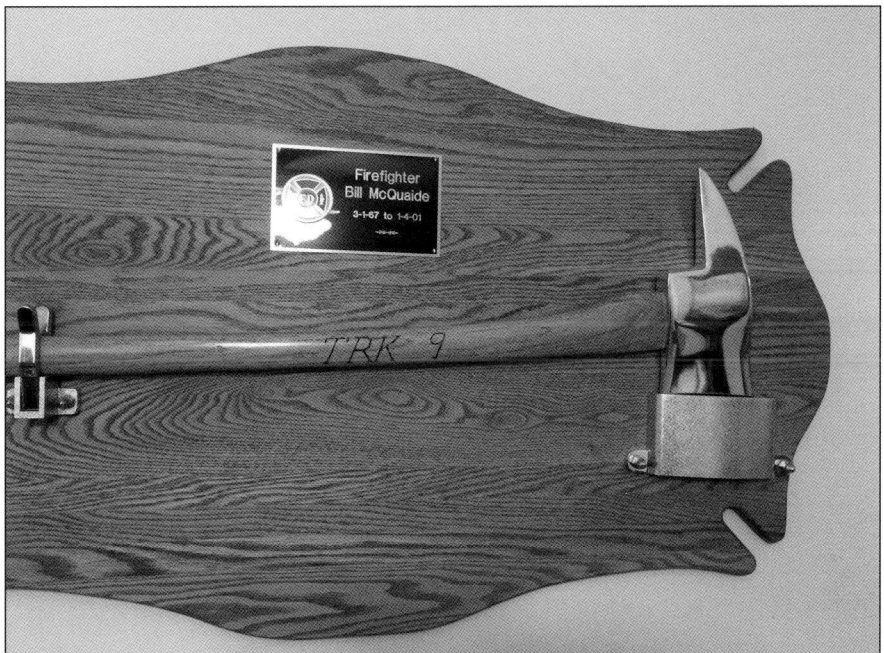

Figure I–2.
My dad's retirement axe

If you're a firefighter, you can picture the glances around the room, the awkward silence as the group struggles to muffle their laughter and retain their professionalism. Looking at each other with imaginary thought bubbles: "Is she for real?" I can't even imagine what would have happened if I hadn't been Bill McQuaide's daughter.

So yes, I learned the hard way. About four classes in, I smartly mustered the courage to ask a participating firefighter for feedback on how I should explain yoga poses. He said, "With as few syllables as possible." I was wise enough to both laugh and then take his advice to heart, and this quote continues to be a favorite I relate in my teacher training course.

Most important, I learned that when firefighters come to yoga class because their back is killing them or their mind won't stop racing at night, they don't want to hear about how yoga is going to help, they just want to experience less pain, whether physical, mental, or both. In other words, get to the point.

Getting to the Point: The Central Questions This Book Answers

Every FireFlex Yoga class is targeted to first responder needs. Getting to that level of specificity, however, takes a complex synthesis of science, deep knowledge of yoga and meditation, and an appreciation of how these practices can work in a traditional warrior culture. This book covers the big issues involved in bringing a program into the firehouse that works for first responders.

These are the two main questions I answer in this book:

- How can yoga practice work as a targeted functional fitness routine to deliver improved movement awareness and prevent a career wracked with injury and pain?
- How can yoga and mindfulness practices work as a mental fitness practice to help firefighters train their brains to manage stress and traumatic injury and promote improved mind-body resilience?

The remarkable advances in neuroscience have made it possible for me to answer the first question, at least as well as a nonscientist can. Quantified results from several years of doing FireFlex Yoga and the heartfelt testimonials from firefighters made it possible for me to answer the second question. The bottom line is that yoga and mindfulness help firefighters rewire their brains so they can take control over their own bodies to move better, think better, handle pain and stress better, and enjoy their personal life and families more. Not bad for rolling out a yoga mat!

Who This Book Is for and How to Use It

This book is for firefighters and the people who want to work with them and understand them better. Individual firefighters can begin practicing some of the poses and mindfulness techniques at home; department chiefs can bring the research and program evaluation statistics to meetings to show how yoga could be incorporated into their existing wellness programs; yoga teachers can learn how to tailor their work for firefighters and other special populations; and counselors, therapists, and support agencies can deepen their understanding of the culture and avoid the typical mistakes nonfirefighters make. Other first responder groups can extrapolate much of the information from the book for their own wellness programs.

This book is organized into six parts, and you can jump in anywhere. I know firefighters are typically kinesthetically driven, so they can go right to part 5 and start doing poses. In fact, doing a little yoga practice before you sit down to read some of the other chapters will clear your mind and thereby ready you to digest the useful information in the rest of the book. And readers will find stories from firefighters in every chapter that are based on interviews I conducted for the book and on the many experiences firefighters have shared with me over the years in my fire family.

In part 1, I explain how the crisis in the fire service is leading to an unprecedented rise in suicides, depression, posttraumatic stress, chronic medical conditions like hypertension and diabetes, and off-the-charts incidents of certain cancers. Firefighters already know this information because they live it every day, but it's critical that the support people who work with them understand more clearly what first responders are up against as their jobs become even more stressful and dangerous.

Just what is yoga? Is my program like hot yoga? How does a "spiritual" practice like meditation belong in the hard-charging first responder environment? What could yoga possibly have to do with resilience? In part 2, I tackle these questions and many more that firefighters and fire chiefs ask me when they want to know if yoga will fit in their organization.

Part 3 is all about the science. Chapter 4 gets into the nitty-gritty of the stress response, especially how it manifests for many firefighters. Chapter 5 packs in a lot of research, but just pick one section that looks interesting to you, such as heart disease or trouble sleeping, and see what the studies say about how yoga and mindfulness are helping. For decision makers who need solid research to make the case for including these practices in their wellness programs, chapter 5 will make your life easier. If knowledge is power, then having a basic understanding of what's happening in your body can give you more control and enable you to manage stress better.

In part 4, I present nuts-and-bolts information for how fire leadership can set up a program like FireFlex Yoga in their departments, including where to have classes, how to set objectives, and how to quantify success, including examples of the measurement tools I use. I present the pre- and postprogram results of five years of data from FireFlex Yoga programs, showing how yoga and mindfulness are improving resilience for firefighters.

Above all, this book is meant to be useful to firefighters, so part 5 invites you to roll out your yoga mat and start practicing. Chapters 8–12 describe the primary sequences used in my typical 10-week program. Each chapter in this part begins with a list of movement objectives, poses, mindfulness practices, and breathing exercises for a particular sequence. Detailed instructions for the poses and exercises are given, along with the most common challenges firefighters come up against, both physically and mentally. Yoga teachers will be able to take these chapters and modify them for their own firefighter yoga classes.

Part 6 focuses on leadership, a subject near and dear to my heart. Over many years working in difficult environments, I've witnessed how learning to be a leader is really the only way to the other side of dysfunction, no matter what the job is. I talk about leadership from a number of perspectives: leading up, leading down, leading our peers, and leading ourselves. Chapter 13 is built around stories about firefighters I admire who are leading the fire service in so many ways, from starting a new initiative to help firefighters deal with depression and suicide to fine tuning the wildfire public alert messaging system.

The final chapter is a yoga challenge. This adapts the Workout of the Day (WOD) that's already very popular with firefighters into a Workout of the Week (WOW). I've done this because I know firefighters will appreciate the additional challenge: five weeks of yoga sequences, including mindfulness meditations. Detailed instructions and photographs are provided so that even if you're a beginner, you'll be able to follow the sequences. Firefighters can practice the sequences at home or in their stations, and yoga teachers can adapt the sequences for their own practices.

It is my profound hope that this book will inspire firefighters to get on the mat and find a way to participate in and benefit from yoga, no matter how low their comfort level may be initially. Because each time a firefighter is able to breathe through a difficult emotion or event and integrate it, they become conscious leaders of their own lives, and the effects ripple outward to the entire community.

The coronavirus pandemic started right as I was finishing this book, and I talked to a few firefighters who are first responders on the front lines. One of their stories opens chapter 13. From what they told me, using yoga and mindfulness to support operating from a place of calm and grace under pressure in high risk and uncertainty is more crucial than ever. #SocialSolidarity!

Part I

The Crisis in the Fire Service

1

Today's Fire Service Needs a Conscious Warrior Culture

On October 13, 2017, with wildfires raging in Northern California, I got a call from Captain Jason Golden of the Southern Marin Fire Protection District (now a Battalion Chief of the Southern Marin Fire Protection District). Would I be willing to lead yoga and mindfulness classes for the families of North Bay firefighters? I knew Golden from teaching yoga in his department the previous year. He told me that the town of Santa Rosa was at the epicenter of the disaster and many of the firefighters who were out on the fireground had just lost their own houses, their families scattered throughout the area seeking refuge. Not only had many of them lost everything, but they were also afraid for their exhausted partners and spouses battling what became known as the Tubbs Fire—at the time, the most destructive wildfire in California history.

I packed a bag, loaded up my car with yoga mats, and (with my yoga instructor friend Carol Day) drove the 81 miles to the Santa Rosa training facility. As we got north of Novato, we drove into a wall of smoke. In every direction, all we could see was gray. There was no sky, no horizon. Carol and I were already coughing and getting headaches, and we were still about 30 miles from Santa Rosa.

At the time of the Tubbs Fire, I had been delivering FireFlex Yoga programs throughout firehouses in Northern California for almost three years. Having grown up in a household of professional firefighters, I thought I knew a thing or two about their dedication and bravery. Nevertheless, what I experienced over the next few days moved me profoundly.

After we got to Santa Rosa I learned that Golden was spearheading a multipronged approach to this unprecedented crisis along with John Bagala, vice president of International Association of Fire Fighters (IAFF) Local 1775; Todd Landau, secretary of Local 1775; and Tom Moran, engineer paramedic and peer support for Southern Marin Fire Protection District. Golden told me, "We set up a command center at the Santa Rosa IAFF Local 1401 Union Hall. Our first objective was making sure the firefighters living in the area were okay and hadn't perished in the fire; second was determining whose house was okay and whose wasn't, and then we had to figure out what people needed."

Realizing they could use geographic information system (GIS) mapping was a major step in making a house-by-house search possible in the midst of chaos, especially as the fires kept growing: "We had the Tubbs Fire, Nuns Fire, Pocket Fire, Atlas Fire, and Mendocino Complex," Golden explained. "Figuring out how to help the community was a huge undertaking and effort by a number of people who came up with a plan and put it into action."

What moved me so much was the kind of leadership I saw by everyone involved. It truly was grace under fire. Not only did IAFF Local 1775 and other San Francisco Bay Area locals have the backs of the firefighters out on the fireground, some working seven to nine days without a break, but they were also caring for their families and for an entire town. "People were looking at their community and seeing it devastated," remembers Golden. "It looked like a nuclear bomb had gone off." The command center became a place where, in Golden's words, "Everyone could relax a little, take a deep breath, know that they weren't forgotten."

On the first day I was there, off-duty firefighters, families, and community members had access to counseling, yoga, massage, chiropractic, food, and children's activities. Eventually, the program included lawyers and insurance experts, all volunteering to help people deal with legal and insurance issues that were coming at them on top of enormous stress and dislocation. More than $500,000 was raised for the firefighters who lost their homes. A warehouse with donated duffel bags full of clothing and essentials was set up so people could simply drop by and pick one up. Golden said the most important question was always, "What do you need?"

My experience was of people coming together in the midst of tragedy to support each other. I was honored to bring yoga and meditation to give people a few moments of peace and a chance to tap into their inner strength and resilience.

The innovative peer support program created by Bagala, Golden, and their colleagues has become a model for future disaster sites. Being a small part of the effort reinforced for me why I love working with firefighters: family isn't just a word to them. When they say they have your back and that of their communities, they mean it in the deepest sense.

The Tubbs Fire and the dozen other wildfires that broke out at the same time weren't contained until the end of October 2017. By then, an estimated 36,432 acres burned, and at least 22 people had been killed in the Tubbs Fire alone. Sadly, the Tubbs Fire was surpassed by the Camp Fire in 2018, which burned 150,000 acres and killed 85 people.[1] While I was writing this book, the 2019 Kincaid and Sonoma County fires ravaged Northern California again, with Santa Rosa barely missing another disaster. Then, in early 2020, as I was finishing this book, the coronavirus pandemic rampaged across the globe. Once again, the courage and dedication of the firefighters, along with police, EMS, sheriffs, chaplains, and the Federal Emergency Management Agency are making headlines in the local and national news. Like the photographs seared into our collective consciousness of heroic rescues by firefighters after 9/11, images of first responders risking their lives are becoming increasingly part of our culture.

Firefighters and other first responders are heroes, no doubt about it. One of the reasons I wrote this book is to shine a light on the cost to the brave women and men who protect us and keep us safe. What goes on behind the scenes and outside the media coverage should concern us all. Physical injuries, cardiovascular disease, cancer, posttraumatic stress disorder (PTSD), depression, relationship difficulties, drug and alcohol abuse, and rising numbers of suicides are some of the issues facing today's firefighters at rates well beyond those for the general population. Firefighting has always been a dangerous and difficult job. Still, as my father always believed, it is one that is tremendously rewarding. "Shannon," he would say to me, "I hope you have the opportunity to wake up every day and look forward to going to work, like I do."

As the fire service changes, so do the demands on our firefighters. Yoga and mindfulness practices can help them to grow and adapt to the changing face of the fire service. That is the heart of this book.

A Day in the Life: The Changing Face of the Fire Service

For firefighters reading this book, you know firsthand much of the information in this section because you live it every day. However, for civilian readers, such as yoga teachers and mental health counselors who want to work with firefighters, this chapter will explain the demands of the job, an understanding of which is crucial to gain the respect of first responders.

Being a firefighter is one of the most demanding jobs—physically, mentally, and emotionally. Here are just a few examples: firefighters must be able to carry unconscious people down flights of stairs, handle a hose that carries 2,000 gallons of water per minute, extract people from mangled cars, break down locked doors, and do all of this safely and quickly because lives are at stake. Cameron Bucek, a fire and EMS clinical educator, tells his students, "You can die. You can be in top shape, but become stressed and dehydrated at the scene as you climb six flights of stairs and carry someone 250 pounds to safety, with all that gear on your back and that heavy suit on."[2]

Fighting fires is only one part of the job, and the nature of firefighting has changed dramatically in recent decades. The number of fire calls has declined, in part owing to improved fire prevention methods, but the fires are more dangerous and harder to fight. In addition, fire departments have taken on many new responsibilities that are taxing resources and demanding even more of firefighters: mental illness, mass shooting events, natural disasters related to climate change, homelessness, and a tripling in the number of medical aid calls over the past 25 years. In fact, many firefighters are EMTs or paramedics.

Civilians are usually surprised to learn that around 70% of dispatched calls in most fire stations are for EMS, and in some districts, this can even be 80% or more.[3] My brother-in-law, a firefighter/engineer in California, told me his department has seen an exponential increase in call volume from 2017 to 2018, from 65,000 to 100,000 calls. His crew constantly responds to the medical needs of a growing homeless population or to fires started in makeshift housing and encampments for this same demographic.

Firefighters are on the front line of social struggles, too—in particular, the opioid epidemic and homelessness often resulting from addiction. A friend of mine who is a public safety administrator says that close to 100% of the homeless in her city are addicted. If you're not a first responder, this might sound impossible, but it's not. According to the Centers for Disease Control and Prevention (CDC), overdose deaths involving opioids were six times higher in 2017 than in 1999.[4] And firefighters are the ones answering those 911 calls.

When I asked Chief Golden if he thought we were reaching the tipping point with 911 calls, he explained to me that in a lot of communities, especially economically disadvantaged communities, the residents don't have doctors. "They use us and the emergency departments as their doctors," he said. These calls don't typically make the news, but the impact on firefighters can be profound.

Cullen Kreider, a fire chief from Redding, CA, told me that in 2019, only 500 out of 15,000 calls were fires. So what exactly are his firefighters dealing with? I work with firefighters, and I still find the crazy juxtaposition of what they do every day hard to believe.

Here's one week: lift assists to put senior citizens back in their beds; decontaminating their equipment and clothing multiple times a day from scabies, lice, and bedbugs; doing CPR on an infant. "It doesn't matter if you've been doing this 30 years or one year," said Kreider. "You can see something, and it can affect you for the rest of your life."

The Traditional Warrior Culture

Obstacle for the modern firefighter

First responder cultures are often steeped in the values of the *traditional warrior* culture, where the hero goes into battle to protect and serve. I've studied this value system from an academic perspective, and I've experienced it firsthand in my family. Advantages of the traditional warrior culture include dedication to community, integrity, incredible courage, stoicism, and duty before self. However, there are also negatives: ignoring signals of pain and fatigue, being unwilling to ask for help, and normalizing being unable to sleep and drinking to excess. My friend Crawford Coates, who wrote *Mindful Responder*, talks about how alcohol abuse is the most outward sign of suffering.[5] The fire service has taken steps to address this through behavioral health initiatives, such as peer support teams, but there is still a stigma associated with being vulnerable and talking about the impact of critical incidents experienced day in and day out.

There are plenty of reasons why the warrior culture is so prevalent. First, the firefighter code of ethics asks firefighters to conduct themselves in a manner that reflects proper ethical behavior and integrity, to serve in a position of public trust, and to do so regardless of any challenging social and economic conditions. How many non–first responders take an oath that says you'll put your life on the line for your community no matter what?

In his deeply insightful book, *What It Is Like to Go to War*, Karl Marlantes describes traditional warrior culture in vivid detail. He explains how combat veterans live with the awareness that death is just around the corner. Soldiers are expected to follow orders and to make life-and-death decisions that can have lifelong repercussions. Nevertheless, we send our youth to fight our wars, Marlantes says, without adequately preparing them for the spiritual and psychological consequences of what they will face. Instead, many will operate in a misguided belief that by embracing the warrior archetype, they can perform their duty and be the heroes they aspire to. They are left thinking that asking for help to process their often traumatic experiences is being weak.[6]

Firefighters and other first responders deal with many of the same issues as soldiers. For example, every time they enter a burning building, the possibility of injury or death is in the back of their mind. They regularly manage traumatic life-and-death situations that most of us will never encounter. Retired Fire Captain Jeff Dill is the founder of Firefighter Behavioral Health Alliance, and he has run a workshop called "Saving Those Who Save Others" since 2011. When I talked to him about why he started the program, Captain Dill talked about the rising suicide rate within the world of firefighters. Putting on the uniform, he explains, creates the belief that "This is how we have to act, this is how the community expects us to act. We cannot show any sign of weakness."

Even while mental health issues have a stigma within the general population, that stigma is magnified within the first responder culture. Karl Marlantes talks about this as the *shadow side* and describes the cost of not dealing with this: "Although we all have shadows, we all have different ones. My own shadow has many masks. I'm a strong man—my shadow is a weak, effeminate whiner. I'm a hard worker . . . I'm not afraid to take on a challenge—my shadow constantly fears failing."[7] In firefighters, I've seen the shadow side manifest as a form of armor; they use rank, expertise, professionalism, and humor to deflect their wounds, physical and spiritual, about being prepared for every challenge. So instead firefighters don a mask of being invincible, superheroes, tough guys and gals who can handle anything and everything—an "I got this" approach to whatever difficult or even traumatic situation they face.

The concept of the shadow side comes from renowned psychologist Carl Jung. He coined the concept in the 1920s to describe the "inferior, unadapted, childish, and grandiose aspect of our unconscious life"—in other words, those parts of our personalities no one wants to admit having. According to Jung, not recognizing and working with our shadow side means denying basic aspects of who we are. On the other hand, learning to understand and incorporate our shadow side can lead to greater self-awareness, more creativity, and more openness to new ideas—a change in attitude that can help us understand more clearly "the wisdom of the wholeness of life, the good and the evil, the light and the dark."[8] Although Jung's ideas have been studied and debated for a century, the idea of the shadow has remained remarkably relevant and has been incorporated into many of the interventions and therapies used to help soldiers deal with PTSD and other occupational stressors. This idea of wholeness, or integration, is basic to understanding how yoga, mindfulness, and other mind-body techniques work to balance that false separation so many of us live with.

For first responders, understanding wholeness and balance is crucial. Firefighters live a split existence. At work, they must be ready to head into any emergency as soon as the call comes in, regardless of whether they feel afraid, unprepared, or exhausted. Then, when the shift is over, firefighters go home to their civilian lives. If they mistakenly follow the traditional warrior code at home, the cost can be huge, sometimes leading to aggressive or violent behavior. Lisa Houle, a defense attorney for first responders, says that domestic violence and driving under the influence (DUI) are two issues she deals with frequently. Houle's defense will often be based on the attempts that first responders make to cope with untreated PTSD.[9] As Marlantes says, "If you don't recognize your shadow sides, you'll be likely to cause a lot of damage trying to do your heroic deeds."

Masculine versus feminine warrior

Many of the qualities prized in the warrior culture are considered masculine, whereas the rejected qualities are considered feminine: strong versus weak, stoic versus emotional, bravado versus vulnerability. At least that's the stereotype that has been operating for generations in the fire service, although my personal experience has been mixed: so many welcoming and open firefighters have jumped in to support yoga in their stations before it was considered acceptable. The champions of the program (named in the Acknowledgments) steered me through a lot of challenges and red tape. I couldn't be doing this without them. Nevertheless, after years of resistance to change, the cultural perception that women are too weak or too incompetent to handle the dangers and grim realities of the job remains prevalent.

The statistics tell a disturbing story. According to a 2018 article in *Emergency Management*, only 4% of firefighters are women. That's below the police and military at 14%, and worse than almost any industry, including construction.[10] Disturbingly, *FireRescue1* has reported that female firefighters have the highest divorce rate of any profession, but male firefighters have one of the lowest![11] How do we account for this strange double standard? According to the article, the moderate to severe discrimination or harassment female firefighters frequently face negatively impacts their home lives.

I talked to my sister, Tracey Oliver, deputy fire marshal of the Santa Clara County, CA, Fire Department, about her take on gender equality in the fire service. In particular, I asked whether, after all the years she's been on the job, she thinks women are cutting it. She said that all six women, including herself, who went through the fire academy together have gone on to successful careers in the fire service, now all in leadership roles. She also explained that women were more heavily scrutinized than men, whether at the academy or in the station, because it was simply assumed that men are able to do the job whereas women had to prove they could.

I've also had some great conversations with male firefighters who were impressed with decisions their female colleagues have made and how emotional intelligence played a big factor. My friend Fire Chief David Dolson told my teacher-training class about a critical incident he responded to where the outcome was positive because of the role his female colleague played. She delivered the perfect combination of professionalism and compassion to settle down a highly agitated patient, which made the delivery to the hospital much easier. Without her, Dolson said, the call could easily have gone sideways.

Even though gender issues are persistent, they are changing because of hard work by fire leadership and the immensely capable and talented women who are proving themselves in the field. Jenn Panko, chief officer of administration at Santa Clara City Fire Department, is actively reaching out to the next generation to increase diversity by recruiting across all demographics. "At this point in my career, I understand the importance of giving back to my profession," Panko explained. "When young girls see me or other women riding in fire trucks, it sends a very powerful message to them that girls can be firefighters. With a group of other female firefighters, I helped to establish a girl's fire camp for high school–age girls so they can get the chance to explore what a career in firefighting is all about. Mentoring female leaders in the fire service is the most current focus given that the fire service is so male dominated and female chief officers are few and far between. Now, seeing women in chief officer–level positions is what is inspiring to me."

The Conscious Warrior

My perspective as a long-time practitioner of yoga and meditation is that focusing on a limited perception of gender will hinder the transformation of the old concept of the warrior culture to one that will work for today's first responders. The preconception that men exhibit only masculine traits and females exhibit only feminine traits is inaccurate and doesn't portray what is really happening in firehouses around the country. It's not about being just masculine or feminine, strong or weak; it's about the multiple aspects of all of us, including our shadow side. If we're afraid of integrating what we consider to be feminine, then we're in danger of numbing ourselves to feelings like love, gratitude, and compassion, as well as depriving ourselves of the deep connections we crave with others. As first responders adapt to the needs of the 21st century, the positive side of the warrior archetype—duty, honor, and courage—will be more indispensable than ever. Yet at the same time, a more realistic understanding of the hero as a person with many faces and dimensions—including the ability to access the feminine, masculine, and shadow sides—is essential.

One passage of the Marlantes's book in particular made me think about the career trajectory of most firefighters, who start out as young adults full of vigor and idealism and try to maintain a healthy life for themselves and their families over 20 or more years of doing a dangerous job. Marlantes is talking about the military, but there are so many similarities:

> The heroic journey can be taken consciously or unconsciously. There's a time in one's life when the unconscious heroic journey is understandable, when one is young and in positions of little authority. The young warriors of the future will still largely perform their heroic tasks unconsciously. It is a part of development, eventually to be outgrown. As warriors grow older, however, and move into positions of power and authority, far more is at stake because their actions affect a far wider field. Because there is more to lose, they will have to perform their heroic acts with full consciousness of the often painful consequences for everyone, including themselves. Many heroic acts of this kind will go unnoticed by society—if not actively denigrated. There will be no medals. This makes such acts far more difficult to do, and therefore even more heroic.[12]

I've had numerous conversations with firefighters about what they want and the changes they would like to see. Many agree that those in leadership positions need to take a more active and vocal stance in supporting firefighter behavioral health, yet those leaders had careers shaped by traditional warrior values. I've also worked with innovative fire chiefs and captains who are leading the way by offering a constellation of programs to support both the physical and mental resilience of their firefighters. I love the description my friend, Battalion Chief Ryan Peters, gives of modern firefighters, who (in his view) can be reflective, insightful, and trusting of the messages they are receiving from their bodies about pain, boundaries, and time to seek support or take a break. Yoga and mindfulness practices can support the development of the conscious warrior.

The conscious warrior is showing up in big and small ways. For example, in one station where I was doing my yoga program, there was a lot of good-natured joking about my being a vegetarian. "Who wants to eat tofu!" was a typical comment. However, I perceived that their humor hinted at a growing interest in eating more healthfully and how that might alleviate problems such as high blood pressure or the extra pounds that can creep up on firefighters given their erratic schedules. I was touched when after the last yoga class they presented me with a fabulous vegetarian meal they had prepared from a book called *Eat Like You Give a F*ck.* Here was humor combined with a willingness to explore new ideas that aren't in the traditional fire service culture—not only did they make me feel accepted, but they were also letting me know that yoga was making a positive difference in their lives.

A Day in the Life

The physical toll

This section describes the physical toll on firefighters. Except where otherwise indicated, the statistics used here are from the National Fire Protection Association (NFPA).[13] Every year, the NFPA puts out a report on firefighter deaths and injuries. The 2017 figures show that across the nation, 60 firefighters died in the line of duty that year, almost half from cardiac arrest. What's good is that this number is down from previous years (a decrease of 5% from 2016), in part because of improved fire prevention methods.

The number of injuries, however, is mind boggling. The NFPA estimated that 58,835 firefighter injuries occurred in 2017, with 24,495 injuries happening at the scene of a fire and the rest during other nonfire events like rescues, vehicle extrications, hazardous materials incidents, and most prevalent, emergency medical calls. The most common injuries included overexertion, strains, sprains, burns, and wounds. In addition, there were 7,345 documented exposures to infectious diseases including hepatitis, meningitis, and human immunodeficiency virus (HIV); there were a further 44,530 documented exposures to hazardous conditions such as asbestos, chemicals, fumes, and radioactive materials. Now imagine that kind of exposure over a 20-year career! Of these injuries, 17% led to firefighters having to take time off. While that might not sound like a big number, that translates to 10,155 incidents in a single year. The NFPA report concludes that "It is not possible to accurately assess the total number of deaths and injuries that have resulted annually due to long-term exposures to carcinogens and physical and emotional stress and strain."

What about the annual economic cost of injuries and illness? The NFPA's 2019 bulletin, "The Economics of Firefighter Injuries in the United States," reported a range of $1.6 billion to $8.4 billion (after dropping the highest and lowest figures).[14] What really struck me is that the number of injuries at nonfire emergencies increased 28% between 1981 and 2017, from 9,600 to 12,240. That number is not surprising given that the number of nonfire emergencies increased 332%! The NFPA suggests that most of this increase is because of medical calls. However, since they don't look at what kinds of medical calls make up these numbers, we can't know for sure how many are due to the drug epidemic and challenges of homelessness.

The pie chart in Figure 1–1 breaks down the types of injuries that happen at the scene of a fire. Interestingly, the almost 50% of injuries caused by overexertion (strains and sprains) and falls, jumps, slips, and trips are precisely those that yoga and mindfulness techniques can help prevent. Notably, these types of accidents also happen at nonfire scene events.

Disturbingly, firefighters are at significant risk for certain cancers. According to the Firefighter Cancer Support Network, firefighters have a 9% higher risk of being diagnosed with cancer and a 14% higher risk of dying from cancer than the general population. These statistics are based on a 2010 study by the National Institute of Occupational Safety and Health (NIOSH). The NIOSH study also identifies specific types of cancer for which the numbers go up dramatically: in particular, firefighters are twice as likely—that is, 100% more likely—to get mesothelioma.[15] The rates vary across the country, with some departments having even higher numbers.

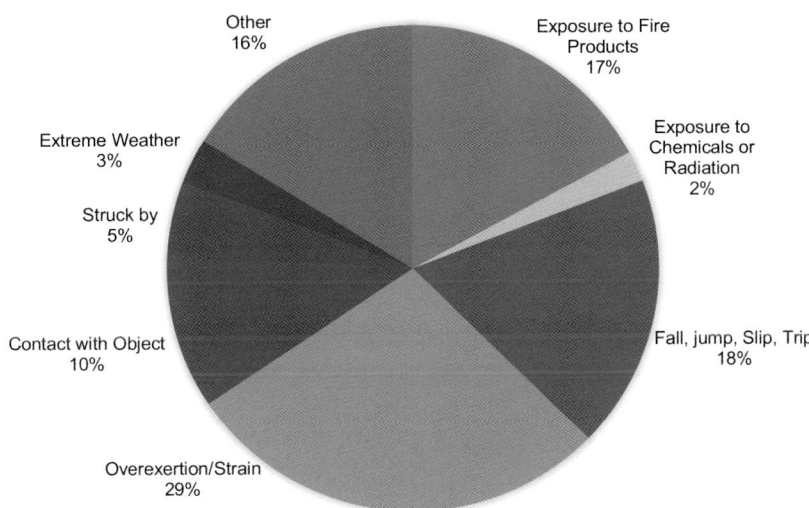

Figure 1-1.
Fireground injuries by cause, 2018
(From *United States Firefighter Injuries*, 2018, NFPA, Richard Campbell, Ben Evarts, and Joseph L. Molis, December 2019)

Heart attacks are the leading cause of death for active-duty firefighters.[16] A 2019 study in the *Journal for Occupational and Environmental Medicine* that looked at the high incidence of cardiovascular disease in firefighters and law enforcement officers reported that the mortality ratio for middle-aged firefighters is 73% greater compared with nonfirefighters. This next quote from the study should be a wake-up call for all of us: "The elevated [cardiovascular disease] risk in firefighters and law enforcement officers could be considered a threat to national security given their importance as first responders to national emergencies."[17] The report is very positive in concluding that interventions in lifestyle can significantly reduce risk factors for cardiovascular disease. In summary, according to the report, a complete picture of duty-related fatalities would also include deaths resulting from cancer, cardiac issues, and stress, as well as other fatalities that were caused by exposures to toxins or the emotional toll of responses.

In the next chapter, I will go into more detail on how these risk factors can be mitigated by yoga and mindfulness techniques in conjunction with other strategies such as healthier eating habits.

The emotional toll

The May 2018 report of the Substance Abuse and Mental Health Services Administration, *First Responders: Behavioral Health Concerns, Emergency Response, and Trauma*, has the latest statistics on mental health and substance abuse issues with first responders.[18] The report estimates that 30% of first responders develop behavioral health conditions like depression and PTSD. Another striking finding is that firefighters often believe that getting mental health support could derail their careers.

I asked Jeff Dill what he thought was happening, and he believes that over time, repeated tragedies can wear down even the toughest heroes. The home page of the website for his organization, Firefighter Behavioral Health Alliance, keeps a running tally of the first responders who take their own lives. He started the tally in November 2010. As of July 4, 2021, 1,381 firefighters, 256 EMTs, and four dispatchers have completed suicide.

The fire service and the media are working together to get the word out to the general public that our first responders are in crisis. WNBC in New York collaborated with the IAFF on a major survey on PTSD in the fire service. Their two-part broadcast in 2018 reached millions of viewers and revealed what's really happening. More than 7,000 IAFF members responded to the survey, with an overwhelming number reporting that stressful or traumatic experiences on the job have affected their mental health: 19% have had thoughts of suicide, 27% have struggled with substance abuse, 59% have experienced family and relationship problems, and 65% are haunted by memories of bad calls.[19] These numbers are well above those for the civilian population.

Even more concerning, 81% of those surveyed said they "feared being seen as weak or unfit for duty if they asked for help." And 71% reported not using services provided by their department for mental health issues. This certainly sounds like the negative aspects of the warrior culture. Of those who did use services, 63% did not find it helpful. Part of the problem, according to IAFF President Harold Schaitberger, is that there are not enough clinicians who understand the fire service.

Conclusion

Reflecting on all the statistics and challenges mentioned in this chapter, how could yoga possibly fit into the fire service, with its embedded warrior culture and distrust of change? As I've discovered after years of working in fire stations, when you dig down beneath the stereotypes, you'll find that yoga complements all aspects of the fire culture.

The rest of this book describes how yoga and mindfulness can support five key benefits for first responders:

- Reduced injuries and improved movement quality
- Reduced chronic and traumatic stress
- Improved cardiovascular health
- Improved quality of sleep
- Increased situational awareness and self-understanding

Part II

East Meets West—Why Yoga Belongs in the Fire Station

2

From Badass Warrior to Savasana

THE BENEFITS OF YOGA FOR FIREFIGHTERS AND FIRST RESPONDERS

War and Peace on the Mat

The reason yoga fits so naturally into the warrior culture is illustrated in the story of the *Bhagavad Gita*. Thousands of years ago, yogi warriors in India found themselves on a battlefield of epic proportions. As he prepares to fight, the hero of the story struggles to understand the central question of *dharma*: how do we perform our duty in the midst of great suffering?

Centuries later, the *Bhagavad Gita* remains a profound description of how to perform our duty, both in the literal sense of actions on the battlefield as in the figurative sense of how we approach the inner struggle—the war within ourselves. Yoga is about both. The Western world is more familiar with Hatha yoga, the popular series of poses and breathing exercises, but yoga is also about mastering the mind.

In one of my favorite interpretations, Steven Pressfield explains how the *Bhagavad Gita* takes the warrior ethos and directs it "inward, employing the same virtues used to overcome external enemies—courage, patience, will, selflessness, the capacity to endure adversity—but enlisting these qualities now in the cause of the inner struggle for integrity, maturity, and the honorable life."[1] Pressfield's book *Gates of Fire* is required reading at West Point and Annapolis and for all officers in the U.S. Marine Corps. It provides training tools for developing the conscious warrior.

Yoga, roughly translated to yoke, means conscious union of mind, body, and spirit. When we intentionally support the body and mind working together, we can harmonize our internal struggle more skillfully and then bring this balance into our work and our relationships with others. In more subtle interpretation, yoga means being on the path to self-knowledge and understanding the pain and suffering in life from a wiser perspective.

This is why yoga belongs in the firehouse. We can't expect first responders to see the level of human tragedy and violence day in and day out without some long-term consequences. They need a framework to process their experiences, one that is tangible and not solely based on faith or religion or requiring allegiance to any other particular belief system. They need a framework that is tactical, visceral, and scientific.

Of course, I don't want to oversimplify. There certainly are differences in the yoga and first responder cultures. The fire service, on the one hand, is very results and outcomes oriented. Their training is a means to an end—fighting a fire, extracting a vehicle, pulling hose, and so on. Yoga, on the other hand, is more process than product. That is, we practice yoga for achievement of greater self-awareness, which is an ongoing process.

A couple times a year, I conduct yoga teacher-training programs using a curriculum developed specifically for working with firefighters and other first responders. One of my favorite parts of the training is when Division Chief David Dolson of the Roseville, CA, Fire Department talks to the students about doing yoga in the firehouse. As head of training for his division and a certified yoga instructor himself, Dolson is the perfect person to talk about the two cultures. This is what he said during one of the training sessions:

> The values in the fire service parallel yoga philosophy: honor, courage, respect, and devotion to duty. Self-awareness in yoga parallels situational awareness in the fire service—we bring ourselves back to those core values and act accordingly to whatever is put in front of us. Yoga practice helps us grow our internal situational awareness and then our professional awareness with each other, with our co-workers, and with everyone we interact with.

The Yoga Continuum: You Decide

The other day, I saw at least 10 publications and advertisements that showed people doing yoga. Beautiful photographs showed stunningly fit people in expensive Lululemon outfits, on beaches or in exotic resorts. The yoga I'm writing about in this book is not that same glossy, packaged version that makes millions every year, with $25 drop-in classes where you can get a kale shake afterward. There's nothing wrong with that version. I'm glad more people are finding out about and experiencing yoga and mindfulness. I've even taught some of those classes! But as a practice that is thousands of years old, yoga offers so much more.

Firefighters can decide where on the continuum they want to practice, from simply getting some physical exercise to going deeper into developing internal awareness and taking steps to experience life more fully and consciously. They can practice yoga in the firehouse or in their living room, with friends or alone. There's no need for fancy outfits.

On one end of the continuum, there is some seriously intense warrior yoga going on. A 2017 study by the RAND Corporation reports that four out of five military health-care facilities in the United States offer yoga. Ex-U.S. Navy SEAL Mark Divine runs Sealfit, one of the most badass programs available to civilians that incorporates yoga and mindfulness techniques. Just watching the videos on his website makes me break a sweat.

This is the attitude I came in with when first implementing my fire station yoga program. I knew that when a lot of firefighters thought of yoga and meditation, they were seeing the glossy, kale shake version. Little did they know that I had a 55-minute power yoga boot camp that would dispel any wrong ideas they might have.

Time for Savasana!

One day, not long into those early days of the program, I was walking into a station to do a class when I heard a blaring message repeated over the station's public address system: "Time for Savasana!" I was thrilled that people were clearly excited about the class, but I couldn't figure out why they were so excited about this particular pose. Savasana isn't one of the really challenging poses. It comes at the end of a class. A rough translation is corpse pose. So what was up?

By the end of class I figured it out. It wasn't that they didn't want to be challenged. Just the opposite: I knew these firefighters; they were always ready for a challenge, and they liked working with their bodies. The technical term for this is that they are *kinesthetically driven*. What I realized was that given the crazy demanding environments in which they work, they were expressing a need for the rest and recovery that Savasana provides. The three to five minutes of quiet time at the end of a class made all the preceding work worthwhile.

That's when I made a decision to incorporate *downtime* throughout fire station classes. I shifted the tempo and goal from being a power workout to being an opportunity to integrate all that is seen, heard, felt, and experienced in a single 24-hour shift. I know this is where the magic of yoga takes place, the integration of body and mind and the development of self-awareness.

As for the Savasana pose in particular, once you get what this pose really does, you understand that it can help balance the nervous system and transform stress. Through the stillness of the Savasana pose, firefighters experience more clearly the impact that the job is having on their lives. Ultimately, practicing yoga bridges the gap between the experience of oneself on the yoga mat and the experience of oneself in uniform, as well as to bridge the distance between the traditional warrior culture to the conscious warrior culture.

Today, there are eight major styles of yoga being taught, from the more gentle Hatha to the more strenuous Ashtanga, or hot, yoga. Some styles incorporate more mindfulness and meditation, others focus more on physical stamina; some are fast paced, others more slow and gradual. My program, FireFlex Yoga, is built on the principles of *interoceptive yoga*—more on that in the next chapters. Whatever the style, the research shows that practicing yoga can bring a number of significant health benefits. In later chapters, I will go into more depth about benefits for firefighters, but this next section gives you a broad overview of what you can expect when you hit the yoga mat.

The Benefits of Yoga for Body and Mind

Those of us promoting the benefits of yoga and mindfulness now have decades of robust research supporting our claims. I'm very happy about this because these practices have often been met with skepticism, even hostility, since their arrival in the United States in the late 19th century. Pictures of yogis with long beards and beads around their necks doing superhuman contortions probably didn't help! The long list of health benefits also seemed hard to believe. How could sitting around with your eyes closed produce anything but a nap? But skeptics are now on shaky ground, given the increasing numbers of studies and medical programs incorporating alternative practices like yoga and mindfulness.

I spend considerable time keeping up with current research, but combing through the thousands of studies is impossible. A search on the PubMed database of the National Library of Medicine using the keywords "yoga" and "low back pain" retrieved 176 matches. There were 710 matches for "yoga" and "anxiety"! In this section and throughout the book, I incorporate the viewpoints of the most reputable medical organizations in the

United States about the benefits of yoga and mindfulness on both body and mind. These experts have reviewed the research, used the practices with their patients and clients, and have the credibility to make the claims. My goal is to present what's most beneficial to first responders.

Let's start with a definition. The Mayo Clinic defines yoga as "a mind-body practice that combines physical poses, controlled breathing, and meditation or relaxation."[2] Pretty much everyone agrees that yoga incorporates these three components, with the ratio varying depending on the style. Based on abundant research, Harvard Health says, "The evidence is growing that yoga practice is a relatively low-risk, high-yield approach to improving overall health."[3] Thus, the Mayo Clinic and Harvard Health agree that the evidence suggests yoga is beneficial for both anxiety and depression. Both list the following as the most well-documented benefits:

- Reduced stress
- Lower blood pressure
- Lower heart rate

In the sidebar, you'll see an impressive list of physical benefits cited by the American Osteopathic Association. This represents great news for firefighters given the number of injuries they suffer and the alarming rise of cardiovascular disorders and behavioral health issues.

> ### Physical Benefits of Practicing Yoga[4]
>
> - Increased flexibility
> - Increased muscle strength and tone
> - Improved respiration, energy, and vitality
> - Maintaining a balanced metabolism
> - Weight reduction
> - Cardiovascular and circulatory health
> - Improved athletic performance
> - Protection from injury

Chronic and acute pain

Some of the most exciting research shows the benefits of yoga for managing pain. The military has been particularly interested because of the effects of the opioid crisis.[5] One report estimated that by 2011, 25%–35% of wounded soldiers were dependent on prescription pain relievers.[6] While the numbers have decreased significantly, probably because of prevention programs by the U.S. Department of Defense (DoD) and Veterans Affairs (VA), pain management continues to be a critical issue.[7]

The military launched several major studies to look into whether yoga and mindfulness could address the problem because surgery and drugs were not working. In 2017, the American Congress of Rehabilitation Medicine published the results of a groundbreaking study on the practicality and effectiveness of an individualized yoga program, called RESTORE (Restorative Exercise and Strength Training for Operational Resilience and Excellence), that was designed to treat chronic lower-back pain in service members and their families using an eight-week series of yoga classes. The results indicated that "RESTORE may be a viable nonpharmacological treatment for low back pain with minimal side effects."[8]

In fact, the U.S. Department of Health and Human Services, the DoD, and the VA are investing $81 million to develop nondrug pain management approaches, including yoga and meditation. Eric Schoomaker, M.D., Ph.D., who served as the 42nd Surgeon General of the U.S. Army, has been on a mission to bring yoga to military health care. In his experience, people who are using yoga to rebuild function and improve pain are not turning to surgery and drugs. Dr. Schoomaker says that "We ought to be frontloading practices such as yoga that focus on function and whole-body wellness—using them offensively and defensively as the first step in preventive care and medical treatment before chronic pain, illness, and drug use become issues."[9] These are strong words from someone from the front lines of the warrior culture.

The important questions to answer for those of us talking to first responders about yoga are:

- Why is the military looking at yoga's ability to promote operational resilience and excellence?
- How can an eight-week yoga program start to bring results like the ones mentioned in the 2017 American Congress of Rehabilitation Medicine study and the many other studies showing similar outcomes?

To answer these questions, the research suggests that yoga helps us perceive stress differently, which helps us to regulate our stress response systems. Being able to modulate our response to stress is the key to reducing heart rate, lowering blood pressure, and easing respiration—those well-documented benefits that play a critical role in mitigating so many of the physical and emotional issues first responders face.

Conclusion: How Do You Strengthen Your Mind?

Most firefighters know how to create a physically strong body, and many stations have fitness rooms with treadmills, top-of-the-line strength training equipment, free weights, and kettlebells. However, when I ask firefighters, "How do you strengthen your mind?" I mostly get blank stares. Because firefighter performance is a balance of both mental and physical fitness, ignoring either one of these facets can be a big liability. Practicing yoga strengthens both.

There is a reason for the blank stares. When Western medicine hundreds of years ago divided mind and body into two separate entities, the practice of treating each separately became the norm. Depression and anxiety were considered mental problems that needed to be fixed by treating the mind. Chronic pain was considered a physical problem that needed to be fixed by treating the body. Unfortunately, behavioral health issues were often disparaged as weaknesses of the mind or of character. Finally, what we've been learning from research over the past 30 or so years is that problems have resulted from ignoring that the whole system works together. As the military is finding out, treating people as one cohesive being is bringing significant benefits in resilience and peak performance.

3

What Does Resilience Have to Do with Yoga?

Resilience: Where Warrior Culture and Yoga Culture Meet

From education to business to the military, everyone wants to develop resilience. The consensus across these diverse groups is that resilience is a critical component of both physical and behavioral health. In fact, Leadership Under Fire founder Jason Brezler suggests that mental conditioning will be just as important as physical conditioning for firefighters. He also points out that the fire service, like other first responder groups, has often approached resilience and mental health in a reactive fashion—after someone is having trouble readjusting after trauma.[1]

Exactly what is resilience? Is it mental toughness, bouncing back after adversity, or something we need only after things get really tough? Moreover, what does resilience mean for first responders?

Here's what the military has to say. The Office of the Chairman of the Joint Chiefs of Staff addressed the changing demands on the U.S. Armed Forces in the "Chairman's Total Force Fitness Framework," released in 2011:

> Given the current demands placed on our forces, a Service member's resilience—ability to withstand, recover, *grow, and adapt* [italics mine] under challenging circumstances—is vital to readiness and mission accomplishment. Without resilience, service members and their families are at risk of burnout, psychological stress, and physical danger due to impaired functional abilities.[2]

The first responder world is heavily influenced by the military. *First Responders: Behavioral Health Concerns, Emergency Response, and Trauma*, a 2018 research bulletin from the federal government, lists a number of studies showing that resilience training (including yoga and meditation) given to first responders including police and firefighters reduced stress and improved performance in the line of duty. The report concluded that "a cooperative effort is needed between organizational leadership and coworkers to establish a work environment that provides adequate training and ensures the resilience and health of first responders by *protecting them from overwork and excessive stress and supporting them in seeking help* [italics mine] when needed."[3]

What does resilience really mean for first responders?

Putting all this together, we're getting closer to a better working definition of resilience. As a first responder, if you have good resilience, then you know how to protect yourself from stress and a crazy schedule, you know how to modulate and bounce back from challenging or traumatic events and are not hesitant to ask for help, and you know how to keep growing and adapting to new situations and new challenges. This kind of resilience calls for both your mind and your body to perform at the highest levels. It calls for you to possess the kind of mindset that sees all kinds of challenges as opportunities to learn—a tall order!

Because yoga and mindfulness work through mind-body integration, they are ideally suited to complement other approaches to resilience. Dr. Madhu Hardasmalani, assistant professor of emergency medicine at the Keck School of Medicine at the University of Southern California, has worked with first responders for years. She explains that building resilience is a principle goal of yoga through "tapping into the power of the mind to help us develop new habits, new ways of relating to the circumstances of our lives, whether that be physical pain, emotional trauma, or just plain stress." Dr. Hardasmalani adds, "All forms of exercise can help us feel better, but yoga is the only form of exercise that isn't fatiguing and helps us connect the three important aspects of resilience: body, mind, and spirit."[4]

Resilience and self-awareness

If yoga is a union of mind, body, and spirit, then what exactly is spirit? Depending on what yoga teacher you talk to, what form of yoga you practice, or your own personal beliefs, it can mean just about anything: universal consciousness, the soul, love, God, or nothing at all. In my program, I talk about spirit as self-awareness because that's one of the most important life skills yoga develops: a conscious recognition of what's really going on in the moment and a knowledge of our own character, abilities, and feelings.

Self-awareness is the key to taking charge of lives, to building the kind of resilience that leads to peak performance. The army considers self-awareness a core leadership capacity and promotes its development to improve a number of functions, including critical thinking and professional development.

Resilience doesn't mean fixing things

Almost every firefighter I work with talks about the emotional pain of not being able to fix things: drug addiction, having to leave children in crack houses, responding to a fire where a family is living in a garage and cooking on a dangerous propane stove, or repeat visits to emergency rooms from "frequent flyers" (the elderly or homeless people without resources who firefighters respond to over and over). These are some of the challenges in the modern fire service. Feeling miserable, discouraged, or frustrated in these circumstances is appropriate. Not reacting or feeling anything is not a sign of resilience.

Yoga and mindfulness techniques don't take away the pain and frustration of feeling helpless, but rather help people to "change their relationship to their circumstances" and get better at managing the natural emotional and empathetic responses that come from witnessing tragedy and hopelessness.[5] Thus, they are valuable tools for coping with the unfixable problems that too often fall on the shoulders of first responders.

How Mindfulness Works

Mindfulness is often considered a kind of meditation. When I use the word meditation in this book, I'm describing a range of practices that quiet the mind. By contrast, mindfulness is a specific practice that brings full attention to the body and mind in the present moment. Check out the sidebar for two popular definitions of mindfulness.

Mindfulness is something we all have the capacity to do. The practice is based on the idea that all of us possess innate wisdom and knowledge we can tap into at any moment. Mindfulness techniques just remind us to do so! The techniques are simple to do, they don't take a lot of time, and many can be done almost anywhere. They include breathing exercises, journaling, visualizations, and paying attention to what's happening in the moment.

Sharon Salzberg, a pioneer of mindfulness in the United States, described mindfulness as those moments when you realize your mind has drifted off and you gently bring it back, with no judgment. This explanation is helpful because it emphasizes how being gentle with oneself is at the heart of mindfulness. It's analogous to driving a car: you don't beat yourself up if your car wanders a bit toward the shoulder; you just bring it back and start again. As you will see, the results of practicing mindfulness can be profound.

> ## Mindfulness
>
> - From Mindful.org: "Mindfulness is the basic human ability to be fully present, aware of where we are and what we're doing, and not overly reactive or overwhelmed by what's going on around us."[6]
> - Jon Kabat-Zinn, a major figure in bringing mindfulness to the West, says mindfulness is "paying attention on purpose, in the present moment, and non-judgementally, . . . in the service of self-understanding and wisdom."[7]

The benefits of mindfulness for body and mind

Jon Kabat-Zinn realized years ago that conducting serious medical research was critical to building an evidence-based case for how mindfulness supports increased clarity and focus, improved productivity, and a host of physical and psychological benefits. He opened the Center for Mindfulness in Medicine, Health Care, and Society (CFM) at the University of Massachusetts Medical School in 1979, and it has become one of the best-known centers for rigorous research and bringing evidence-based mindfulness programs to doctors, staff, patients, and the public. One of CFM's most popular programs, the eight-week Mindfulness-Based Stress Reduction (MBSR), has been given to more than 24,000 people. The results are impressive, with MBSR participants reporting 38% reduction in medical symptoms, 43% reduction in psychological and emotional distress, and 26% reduction in perceived stress.[8] Here's the impressive list of conditions that have been addressed through their mindfulness program:

- High blood pressure
- Heart disease, including heart rhythm disorders and coronary artery disease

- Digestive conditions, including irritable bowel syndrome, acid reflux, and peptic ulcers
- Lack of sleep
- Obesity
- Headaches
- Backaches
- Anxiety
- Depression

Autopilot and negativity bias

Why aren't more people practicing mindfulness? Part of the problem is that staying open—being present and paying attention without being judgmental or interpreting events in a certain way—is difficult. We have stressful jobs, challenging interpersonal relationships, and constant demands on our time and energy. In response, it's easier to go on autopilot—not thinking too much and distracting ourselves from difficult thoughts and feelings or physical pain. However, the research on the negative consequences of continually defaulting to autopilot is mounting. As one study puts it, autopilot can become "our default mode of operating whereby we sleep-walk into our choices. It has seeped into more and more areas of our lives and relationships, making us feel out of control."[9] Moreover, living on autopilot increases the tendency humans have toward negativity bias, with potentially dire consequences for first responders.

Our brains are hardwired to react more strongly to negative stimuli. This phenomenon is called *negativity bias* and probably evolved to keep us alive by alerting us to danger. In modern life, negativity bias means we're more attracted to negative news, negative thoughts, and negative habits. If we get into the habit of letting our attention wander to avoid what might be unpleasant feelings happening in the moment, we can end up thinking about things that are *even more* unpleasant. The process becomes habitual: we go on autopilot, not conscious of our negativity bias, and the accumulation of negative thoughts starts affecting our relationships, our jobs, and our health. Constant negative thoughts shape the way we interpret what's happening to us, which can limit our worldview. For firefighters, the costs can be even higher. I hear so many troubling stories from firefighters about how they feel trapped by a recurring loop of negative thoughts and images from previous incidents, leading to problems at home such as loss of sleep and often cause a general feeling of exhaustion—a hallmark of low resilience.

Yoga and mindfulness practices can make firefighters aware that common attitudes from the traditional warrior culture—dismissing pain, avoiding feeling fear or sadness, or covering up strong emotions with jokes or bravado—might be reflexive habits from living on autopilot. Jeff Dill, founder and director of the Firefighter Behavioral Health Alliance, talked with me about what happens when firefighters put on the uniform and feel they have to act only in ways that conform to stereotypes of hero behavior. Dill remarked, "What amazes me is that in 10 years of doing this work *no one* has said to me, 'You know, Jeff, firefighters seem to be struggling with anger issues and addiction issues.'"

Interoception

Mindfulness strengthens our ability to move from autopilot to more self-regulation and conscious decision-making through the process of *interoception*. Interoception is a fancy word for internal perception. In his workshops, Jeff Dill refers to the process as an "internal size-up." One common definition talks about how the nervous system "senses, interprets, and integrates signals originating from within the body, providing a moment-by-moment mapping of the body's internal landscape across conscious and unconscious levels."[10]

Think of it like a gigantic network of receptor cells inside your organs and skin that passes information—10 megabytes per second—to the parts of the brain that are responsible for making sense of it. Interoception is like an internal neuro-biofeedback system teaching us how to regulate our bodies and minds.[11]

Fleet Maull, Ph.D., a 45-year practitioner of mindfulness and the founder of the Prison Dharma Network, says that when we focus, our brains move from the busy, noisy default-mode network to the task-positive brain. Why does this matter? Maull talks about the growing research showing that improved interoceptive awareness enhances our ability for physiological and emotional self-regulation and deepens our resilience, immune system, and overall health and well-being.[12] In fact, current research suggests that "well-being is deeply rooted in the body, a continuous flow of feelings denoting comfort or distress."[13]

Interoceptive yoga

Interoceptive yoga is the foundation of my program. We increase interoception when we consciously bring our awareness to the sensations in our bodies. For example, yoga poses produce sensations in our legs, back, and shoulders. Some of these sensations might be uncomfortable. In fact, we might not be able to complete a particular pose right away. When we focus on these sensations, using the breath and mindful awareness, and meet them with curiosity rather than judging what we're feeling or comparing ourselves to others, we increase our capacity to experience and understand physical sensation. Over time, learning to simply "be" with what we're feeling increases our *window of tolerance*— the level and amount of stress we can optimally handle.[14]

It becomes empowering to know that we're not going to be overwhelmed forever by strong or even traumatic sensations or experiences. This is how firefighters become great leaders under pressure. Being vulnerable and open is the definition of courage. It's the conscious warrior in action.

Faulty predictions: Are you sure you're in danger?

This interoceptive feedback loop can get derailed, though. Not surprisingly, trauma and chronic stress stand out as key disruptors. Soldiers and first responders who are exposed to trauma, for example, can become hypersensitive to certain stressors, and their interoceptive cells send signals to the brain that the body is under attack, even when it isn't. The messages coming back from the brain can cause the same feelings of profound fear that happened during the original event.[15]

Researchers are now beginning to map areas of the brain, particularly the insula and the anterior cingulate cortex, where this kind of reaction can become a pattern and interoceptive cells actually start to predict the wrong outcome based on past experience.[16] This is a habitual experience for people with PTSD. It may also be driving serious behavioral health issues such as depression, drug addiction, and intractable pain. In fact, continuing discoveries into how interoception works promises the development of targeted drug therapy that can address specific spots where signals get disrupted and messages derailed.[17] Check out the sidebar for how the U.S. Marines are working with interoception and mindfulness as preventative strategies for increasing trauma resilience in soldiers.

Resilience Training

In 2014, a group of U.S. Marines who were preparing for deployment to Afghanistan took part in a study to see if mindfulness training could increase their mental resilience to trauma by improving their ability to process interoceptive distress. The marines practiced a specific form of mindfulness—mindfulness-based mind fitness training—that was designed by a former U.S. Army officer with years of training in mindfulness. The program comprised 20 hours of mindfulness training over eight weeks. Based on their performance during stress tests and brain scans, the marines who participated showed a significant reduction in activity of the right anterior insula and the anterior cingulate cortex. These are key areas of the brain that take in interoceptive signals, process them, and send out the messages and feelings that can get disrupted by high levels of stress. These results support the hypothesis that mindfulness "may serve as a training technique to modulate the brain's response to negative interoceptive stimuli, which may help to improve resilience."[18]

Just Three Minutes a Day

Here's a mindfulness practice you can start with: for the next week, when you arrive at the station and turn the car off, take a minute to notice your breath, feel your body, and ground yourself. After your shift is done and you get home, turn the car off and take a moment to do the same grounding practice. This easy exercise can help you transition from on duty to off duty.

What simple ideas: being less judgmental, being more present. Simple, not easy. Yet just like building your physical strength, your mental strength, resilience, and internal situational awareness comes with practice. And one of the most valuable benefits from increasing mental strength is developing a more open mindset.

Developing a Growth Mindset

It's almost 9 a.m. when I pull into the parking lot behind the firehouse where I'm about to teach a yoga class. I see one of the firefighters—I'll call him Tom here—walking toward my car with a smile on his face. Tom is one of the firefighters who (from the beginning) wasn't afraid to try yoga, as he thought it could help him do his job better.

We roll out the yoga mats on the dayroom floor and begin practicing with the other firefighters in the station. About halfway through the class, a call comes in, which was pretty common at this firehouse because of its proximity to the busy downtown. Everyone jumps up and leaves, letting me know that it's a medical call and they'll probably be returning shortly. I agree to wait.

After about 25 minutes, I hear the ventilation system kick on in the apparatus bay, an indication that the engine is returning to the station. A few minutes later, with their turn-outs peeled off and dressed in their department-issued shorts and T-shirts, they make their way back to the mats. Tom, who's excited to resume the class, turns to me and says, "Shannon, you're not only helping us, you're helping the community we serve."

I'm touched, and ask him why he's saying this. "We just responded to a call from one of our frequent fliers," he explains, "and I found myself being much more patient and kinder to this individual. Before yoga I would have been annoyed and impatient—just trying to get through the call as quickly as possible." He was excited to experience this shift in his mindset and told me it's happening a lot more often, and it's making him more engaged with his life, more curious, more compassionate, and less cynical.

Most firefighters who start practicing yoga will start noticing that for the first time in decades, they feel their bodies relax and back and shoulder pain decrease. Many report having the best night's sleep in years after using some of the breath practices to fall back to sleep after a night call. But in the beginning, few can verbalize the effect yoga has on their *mindset*—the way they view the world. This shift in viewpoint is one of the great benefits of mindfulness techniques.

One helpful definition of mindset is the collection of beliefs and thoughts that make up the mental attitude, inclination, habit, or disposition that predetermines a person's interpretations and responses to events, circumstances, and situations. So our mindset is pretty important to every part of our lives.

Growth versus fixed mindset

Carol S. Dweck, Ph.D., is a professor of psychology at Stanford University and one of the world's leading researchers in the fields of personality, social psychology, and developmental psychology. After 30 years of research, she developed the concept of *growth* and *fixed* mindsets to describe how one person can see opportunity everywhere and believe they can change while others see themselves and their abilities as pretty much set in stone. How we view ourselves and our abilities, according to Dweck, can profoundly affect how we live our lives and whether we achieve our potential. In her best-selling book, *Mindset: The New Psychology of Success,* she gives this great example: one person shows up to a new job and realizes they don't know how to do something. They're devastated. The other person shows up to a new job and realizes they don't know how to do something—yet. It's the "yet" stage of mind that allows us to be more creative, more open to new ideas, and less afraid of trying something different.[19]

If we're stuck in a chronically negative mindset, feeling victimized by life—whether it's from the leadership at our organization, cliques at the station, or the responsibilities of everyday life—we feel little power, or *agency,* in our life. When we can see life differently, we can start to live life differently.

The practice of yoga and mindfulness can help us to achieve a more open and flexible growth mindset. Once we have the tools, we can start consciously shifting our mindset into one we choose rather than being on autopilot. That doesn't mean trying to be positive all the time. Intense emotions of grief, anger, and despair are part of being human, particularly for first responders. Learning to have a growth mindset lets us live life more on a continuum: experiencing all the emotions in life, but a life we have more control over.

Conclusion

Yoga and meditation are outside most firefighters' comfort zone. Learning how to be okay with feelings of disappointment at not being able to complete a pose or struggling to relax or focus the mind for just a single breath is not easy, and many firefighters have to overcome feelings of inadequacy at not being perfect right off the bat. However, by sticking with the discomfort, you increase your confidence and resilience to adapt and manage difficult situations. Your window of tolerance for stress will grow.

In the next chapter, I will explore the science behind the concepts: how the mind-body system works and how unmanaged stress can cause a cascade of negative effects on our minds and bodies. Our brains are being shaped all the time, knowingly or unknowingly. The good news is that you can take steps right now to encourage a growth mindset—to stay open to the many ways you can listen to your body and train your mind.

Part III

The Science behind Yoga and Mindfulness

4

How Yoga Reduces Chronic Stress and What That Means for Your Job and Your Life

Are You Using a Backpack to Manage Your Stress?

A firefighter in one of my classes suffered a heart attack before he was 30 years old. Another would check his pulse every time the bells went off because he was so concerned about having a fatal heart attack. He eventually moved to one of the slower stations at his department to finish his career. Almost every firefighter I know talks about having serious trouble sleeping.

After class one day, one firefighter told me about what he calls his metaphoric "backpack." In this backpack are all the problems and feelings he carries around with him all the time: calls he can't ever forget, such as the baby he found drowned in the pool; fights with his wife that drain him emotionally; constant worry about performance and perceived failures. He said at one point the backpack got so heavy it felt like he couldn't put one more item in it. These are the stories that keep me going into firehouses every day and rolling out the yoga mats.

Yoga and meditation are not panaceas. The daunting array of issues facing first responders calls for a combination of solutions, including medical intervention, behavioral health support, exercise, and a healthy diet. Still, as I show in this chapter, chronic stress is at the root of many of the medical conditions that plague first responders, and mind-body approaches like yoga and meditation are particularly good for managing stress.

This is the "how" chapter. In chapter 2, I talked about the benefits of yoga and meditation, and in this chapter I lay out the science behind how they work. You'll learn the latest and best research and the most exciting discoveries in neuroscience on how yoga and meditation can help you not only reduce stress, but transform it into the building blocks for better body and mind resilience. This is research you will want to incorporate into your own presentation to petition your department for more mind-body resources.

Stress—the Good and the Bad

Most of the talk I hear around fire stations about stress is indirect: Who wants to admit that stress is impacting their life, health, or performance? The reality is that stress isn't all bad. In other words, not all stress is bad. In fact, our body handles *stressors*—that's the medical terminology—all the time, with relatively little trouble. The next time you climb several flights of stairs and start breathing faster, that's your body stepping up to handle stress, first by delivering more oxygen to enable you to breathe faster, then bringing your breathing back to normal once you get to the top. When you go outside on a cold day and start shivering because you haven't dressed warmly enough, that's your body producing more heat to bring your internal temperature back to 98.6 °F.

Homeostasis

When you stop and think about it, the ability of our bodies to handle the sheer number of everyday stressors and keep humming along is astounding. An intricate web of feedback loops between our brain and inner organs is always working to maintain *homeostasis*—the state of internal balance and wellbeing that's necessary to keep us alive. To give you an idea of what happens if homeostasis fails, imagine your computer getting infected with the latest malware virus: the rogue agent multiplies, traveling throughout the system and disrupting your computer's ability to operate, maybe even bringing it to a crashing halt. If you've ever experienced the blue screen of death, you know. In the body, homeostasis is controlled by the autonomic nervous system, which manages key functions like body temperature, heart rate, blood sugar, breathing, and blood pressure. The essential *fight-or-flight* response is within the domain of the autonomic nervous system.

The key idea here is that short-term stress is usually not a problem for our autonomic nervous system. Even acute stress, the kind that alerts us to possible danger and can save our lives, is typically handled pretty easily. Consider when someone cuts in front of you while you're driving a vehicle, even with the lights flashing and the siren blaring: your autonomic nervous system jumps into action, turning on the fight-or-flight response so you can quickly hit the brakes. Once the incident is over, you return to normal, or homeostasis. If you can't stop being angry at the jerk who cut in front of you, your body continues to respond to the event, turning acute stress into longer-term stress.

Other examples of good or appropriate stress include the kind that motivates us to try something new, going beyond our comfort level and reaching for a goal we set for ourselves, or to take a stand for those things and people we value. According to the American Institute of Stress, psychologists refer to this as *eustress*, what we feel when we feel excited: "Our pulse quickens and our hormones surge, but there is no threat or fear."[1] This type of stress can be exhilarating and produce a number of positive benefits, such as increased confidence and fulfillment, maybe a promotion, even falling in love!

Chronic stress

When stress is unresolved, though, it becomes chronic. The body's fight-or-flight system stays on or keeps being triggered by certain situations. Trauma can lead to chronic stress, even PTSD, but so too can relationship problems, financial distress, work overload, even a bad diet, if it lands outside your window of tolerance.[2] Division Chief David Dolson told me the typical call volume for the city of Sacramento's busiest fire stations is 40 calls in 48 hours. He shared a grim story of medics in the station passed out on the kitchen table from exhaustion, with empty cans of energy drinks lying about. Check out the sidebar for a list of common signs that indicate you might be suffering from chronic stress.

More worrying, the research is now clear about the link between stress and the rise of chronic diseases and disorders. These conditions affect first responders at much higher rates than the general population, including heart disease, anxiety, depression, and addiction.[3] An article in *Cell Biology* sums up the problem as "failures of homeostasis."[4]

Signs of Chronic Stress

- Angry outbursts
- Anxiety
- Chest pain
- Drug or alcohol abuse
- Exercising less often
- Fatigue
- Feeling overwhelmed
- Headache
- Muscle tension or pain
- Overeating or undereating
- Restlessness
- Sadness or depression
- Sleep problems
- Social withdrawal
- Stomach upset

The Stress Response System: The Superpower That Needs Supervision

The fight-or-flight mechanism is a superpower. In less than a second, your body can produce enough adrenaline and direct it to the right spots so you can jump out of the way of an oncoming car before you even know what you're doing. It can give you the extra energy and intense focus you need to get up in front of a crowd and deliver an important speech or lead your company on the fireground.

This stress response system is controlled through an elaborate mind-body communication loop led by the brain, via the autonomic nervous system and the endocrine system. Figure 4–1 shows that the autonomic nervous system has two parts: the sympathetic nervous system and the parasympathetic nervous system. Basically, this entire chapter is the story of the ongoing tug-of-war between these two systems. The sympathetic nervous system initiates the stress response, and the parasympathetic nervous system brings the body back to homeostasis. The two systems are often referred to as the gas pedal and the brake. Simply visualizing what could go wrong if either system doesn't work correctly should give you the picture of why they need to play well together.

How it works

This section presents a short version of how the stress response system works. I've concentrated on the key spots where things most commonly go awry. These are the spots where yoga and meditation are especially effective.

When you're faced with acute stress, either physical or psychological, your body sends the relevant sensory data—what you are seeing or hearing—to the amygdala. The amygdala is the part of the brain that controls emotions. Its main job is threat evaluation and survival. The amygdala is critical in the development of PTSD. It analyzes the input and sends a distress signal to the hypothalamus. The hypothalamus is the command center that communicates with the rest of the body through the autonomic nervous system.

Next, the hypothalamus activates the sympathetic nervous system, triggering the fight-or-flight response. Nerve pathways in the sympathetic nervous system signal the adrenal glands to start pumping certain stress hormones: adrenaline causes your heart

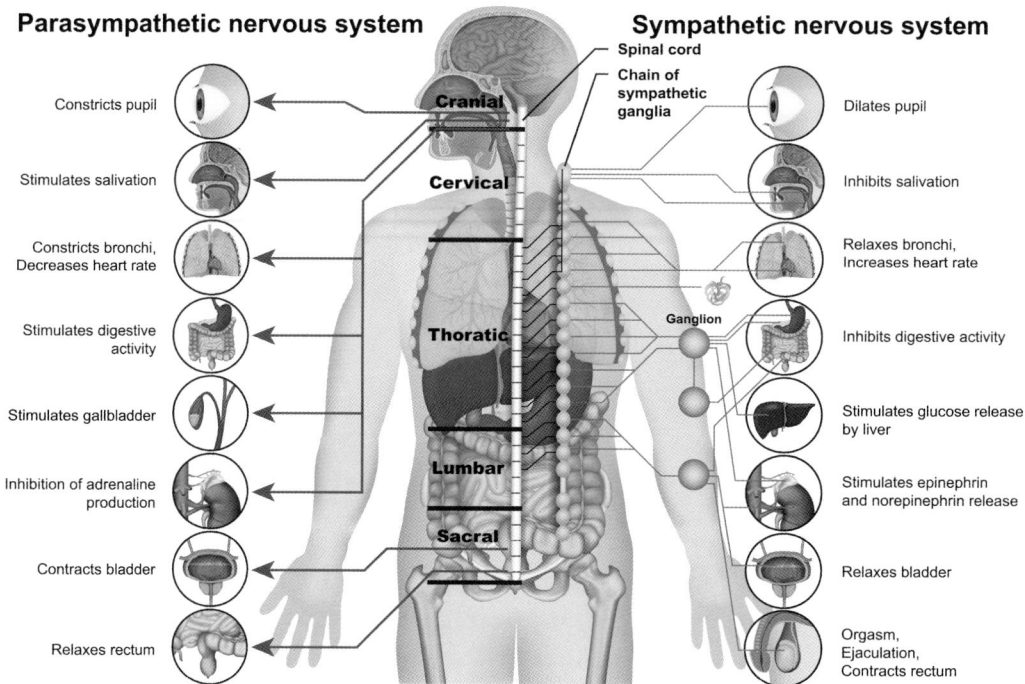

Figure 4–1.
The sympathetic and parasympathetic nervous systems

rate to quicken, your blood sugar to increase for extra energy, your muscles to tighten to either fight or run away, and your breathing to get faster so you have more oxygen. Nonessential systems such as digestion and the immune system shut down to conserve energy. Norepinephrine causes your blood vessels to constrict so our blood pressure rises. You're now ready to deal with the danger.

This cascade of reactions happens instantaneously. Then the second stage kicks in to get you ready for the long game.

Hypothalamic-pituitary-adrenal axis: command central

When the hypothalamus gets information that the danger is ongoing, it activates the feedback system comprising the hypothalamus, the pituitary gland, and the adrenal glands, collectively known as the *HPA axis* (fig. 4–2). This network is one of the most crucial links in the development of chronic disease and behavioral health issues, particularly cardiovascular disorders, depression, and PTSD.

The HPA axis initiates a flood of additional hormones, with *cortisol* being a major player. Known as the stress hormone, elevated levels of cortisol keep the sympathetic nervous system on high alert—in other words, keeping the pedal on the gas so you can continue to handle the crisis. Once the danger is over, your parasympathetic nervous system kicks in, applying the brakes before any damage is done to your body: cortisol and other hormones drop to normal; your heart rate, blood pressure, and breathing return to normal, digestion and immune systems kick back into gear; and your whole system returns to homeostasis. Therefore, keeping the HPA axis in balance, particularly controlling cortisol, is a major part of keeping your body and mind healthy.

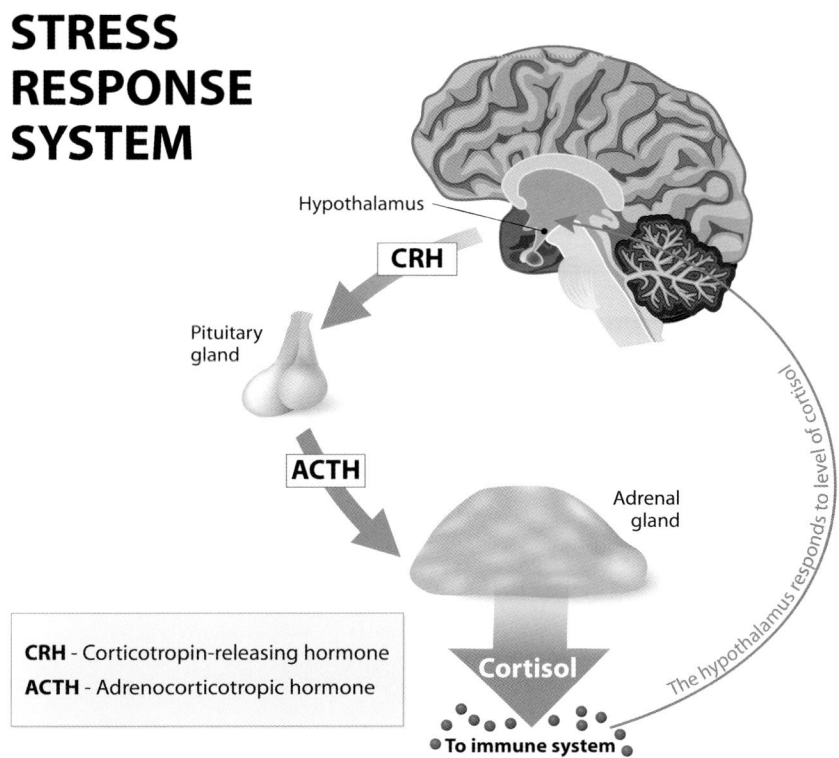

STRESS RESPONSE SYSTEM

Hypothalamus

CRH

Pituitary gland

ACTH

Adrenal gland

CRH - Corticotropin-releasing hormone
ACTH - Adrenocorticotropic hormone

Cortisol

To immune system

The hypothalamus responds to level of cortisol

Figure 4–2.
The HPA axis and cortisol

The negative effects of inflammation

Cortisol, the wonder hormone that can save our lives, can become a key contributor to chronic disease if there's a failure of homeostasis. The HPA axis keeps track of how much cortisol is in the body, increasing and decreasing levels appropriately. However, chronic stress interferes with this balance. If your HPA axis keeps getting signals that the emergency is still on, it just keeps pumping more cortisol. The result is chronic inflammation—one of the major culprits in many diseases.[5]

The Mayo Clinic is blunt about this threat: "The long-term activation of the stress-response system and the overexposure to cortisol and other stress hormones that follows can disrupt almost all your body's processes."[6] This puts you at increased risk of many health problems, including any or all of the following:

- Anxiety
- Depression
- Digestive problems
- Headaches
- Heart disease
- Sleep problems
- Weight gain
- Memory and concentration impairment

If you're a first responder, the consequences of chronic stress are even more concerning because the HPA axis gradually becomes less and less able to maintain balance. An article in *Comprehensive Physiology* explained that "proper control of the stress response is of critical importance, as inappropriate or prolonged HPA axis activation is energetically costly and is linked with numerous physiological and psychological disease states."[7]

Sleep deprivation and caffeine and alcohol consumption also contribute to high cortisol levels, and 20 years of research shows that an out-of-whack HPA axis is associated with problematic alcohol use and dependence.[8] I've been hanging out with firefighters my entire life, and many of them drink coffee to stay awake during long and erratic work shifts. Some drink alcohol to try and downshift the nervous system to reduce anxiety and cope with the demands of the job. However, research shows that increased alcohol consumption can actually increase anxiety.[9] This feedback loop represents a classic "chicken or the egg" causality loop, as the negative effects of stress just keep reinforcing each other.

I talk a lot about the negative aspects of cortisol and inflammation in this chapter, and I want to end this section by clarifying that problems happen when they're out of balance. Still, on the positive side, inflammation is essential for the body to heal itself from disease, injuries, and wounds. The next time you get a shot of cortisol at the doctor's office, you can thank this stress hormone for reducing the inflammation in your painful joint.

Parasympathetic Nervous System: The Vagus Nerve Holds the Keys to the Kingdom

What is your parasympathetic nervous system doing while your sympathetic nervous system is stuck in fight-or-flight mode and the car is careening down the road? It's struggling to put the brakes on. It's still functioning, of course, because you'd be dead otherwise! Imagine your blood pressure going up indefinitely. But the ongoing tug-of-war between these two mechanisms is supposed to maintain a *yin-yang* harmony marked by homeostatic balance. Instead, one side is winning.

Nevertheless, knowledge is power. Once you understand what's happening with an overactive sympathetic nervous system, you can take action to support your parasympathetic system in putting on the brakes.

Often referred to as the *rest-and-digest* or *tend-and-befriend* response, the parasympathetic nervous system is not only vital for recovering after stress but also regulates a number of essential functions including our mood, immune system, digestion, breathing, and heart rate. It promotes healing and repair and restores energy reserves for when we need them for the next fight-or-flight situation.

Importantly, one of the only ways to access the parasympathetic system—and thereby calm down the stress response system—is through the *vagus* nerve, which is the driving force of the parasympathetic nervous system. It's one of the longest nerves in the body and runs from the base of our brain through the neck and chest to the stomach, with an impressive network of branches and nerve fibers that send messages back and forth from the inner organs and to the brain. It's also the main connection with our immune system. Thus, getting accurate input about the state of our heart, lungs, digestive system, and liver all depend on signals from the vagus nerve. Check out Figure 4–3 to see just how impressive it is.

If you're a first responder, I can't emphasize enough how valuable this knowledge is. Messages from the vagus nerve will give you the first clues about what's going on in your body. For example, the gut passes messages via the vagus nerve. So if you're consciously paying attention to your body, as happens during a yoga class, you might sense your gut letting you know that something isn't quite right; this could manifest as a sense of anxiety, or you might get sick to your stomach, or you might feel your heart racing, tightness in your hip, or your thoughts racing. Once you have this awareness, you can send messages back via the vagus nerve letting your brain know to take action. Maybe relax your abdomen, slow your breathing, relax your hip muscles, or redirect your mind from worrying to agency. It's this process of redirecting your mind so that you can control your stress response and how you manage your pain, your relationships, and your life. You can turn toward difficulties and painful situations with confidence, not bravado, and with conscious awareness. It's robust internal situational awareness!

There is a catch, though. So far, the most effective ways we know to stimulate the vagus nerve are through exercise and breathing techniques or inserting a pacemaker-like device in the chest. In one example of how big a deal this is, as late as 1998, scientists thought

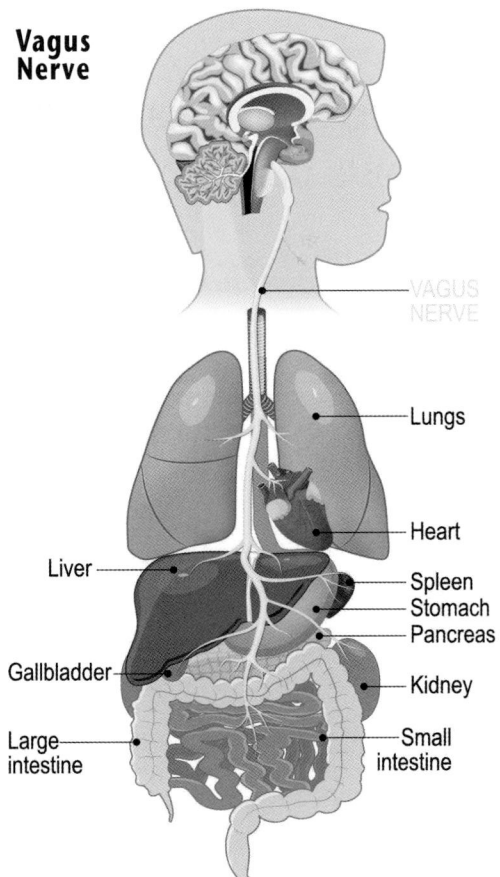

Figure 4–3.
The vagus nerve

that it was impossible for nerves to communicate with the immune system. That was the year neurosurgeon Kevin Tracey performed the first operation showing not only that it was possible to stimulate the vagus nerve through electric impulses but also that doing so significantly reduced inflammation. Given the excitement in the medical field about the role of inflammation, the race was on. A new field of study, bioelectronics, has been directing millions of dollars into developing microregulator implants that deliver electric impulses to stimulate the vagus nerve to treat illness and reduce the need for medication. "Get the nervous system to tell the body to heal itself," is how one reviewer described the new technology.[10]

Yoga and meditation, by contrast, have been using the breath to deliver electrical impulses to the vagus nerve for thousands of years. No surgery needed. Only bringing conscious attention to the mind-body system to get it to heal itself. *Diaphragmatic breathing*, also known as slow abdominal breathing, is something you can do anytime and anywhere to instantly stimulate your vagus nerve and get your neurotransmitters firing to calm your stress response. Scientists from Stanford University think they might have figured out how this happens. They have identified a cluster of neurons that appears to connect different kinds of breathing to different states of mind. So by taking slow, deep breaths, you trigger a response in your brain that leaves you feeling calmer and more relaxed.[11] If you want to try it yourself, check out chapters 8–12 for breathing exercises.

Yoga and meditation are not magic bullets. New technologies like microregulators, for example, are starting to show exciting results, especially in helping serious immune diseases like clinical depression and rheumatoid arthritis. Still, as complementary approaches to overall wellness programs, yoga and meditation can play significant roles in supporting first responders.

Conclusion

Stress is a fact of life. But developing internal situational awareness will help you manage it better and use it for growth. So remember this the next time you think you're too busy to get on the mat!

Don't just take my word for it. The studies highlighted in the next chapter present the evidence. I've chosen only those studies that are most valuable for first responders. It's been thrilling to read so many studies done by some of the most prestigious institutions in the world, all showing how yoga and mindfulness work.

5

Take Heart

HOW YOGA AND MINDFULNESS MITIGATE CHRONIC DISEASES AND DISORDERS

Why You Should Read This Chapter

Cardiovascular disease, depression, anxiety, PTSD, sleep disorders, addiction, cancer, and chronic pain: acute and chronic stress are implicated in each of these threats. If you're a firefighter or other first responder, then you're at greater risk than the general public because of the daily emotional and physical stressors of the job.

You should read this chapter because the main message is positive—there's plenty you can do to prevent or mitigate the negative effects of stress. The concepts explained in chapter 4—the autonomic nervous system, homeostasis, the HPA axis, cortisol, and the vagus nerve—are explained in this chapter in terms of not only how they are the keys to understanding these diseases and conditions but also how yoga and mindfulness can be highly effective interventions for first responders. You'll also get a better appreciation of the science behind how yoga and mindfulness positively affect the parts of the brain responsible for awareness, resiliency, emotional intelligence, and energy management.

I'm a huge supporter of healthy eating, aerobics, and other forms of exercise, as well as an advocate for the role of counseling and medication in managing chronic stress. These components of maintaining a healthy lifestyle are outside the scope of this book, but I want to emphasize that yoga and mindfulness practices are great complements to any departmental wellness program, and they are accessible, affordable, and empowering.

The studies mentioned in this chapter come from evidence-based research from respected peer-reviewed journals. I'm not a neuroscientist or neurobiologist, but I've relied on the brilliant scientists and doctors who make their research easy to understand and relevant. And I don't use any word I can't pronounce! Well, except for cytokines (I had to look it up). But they are key players in the connection between the stress response and illness. I had already become familiar with the research on cytokines and inflammation before the onset of COVID-19, so the "cytokine storm" I kept reading about that was happening with very ill patients made a lot more sense to me.

There's a sense of empowerment that comes from having a basic understanding of the most important functions of our mind-body. Practicing yoga without knowing how it works is fine—you'll get a lot of benefits. Practicing yoga with some understanding of how it works can be transformative. So read this chapter.

Cardiovascular Disease

The hidden role of inflammation

In chapter 4, I talked about inflammation as one of the results of a stress response system in overdrive. Inflammation, in particular, is one of the main culprits in a number of the diseases and disorders that affect firefighters. Mounting evidence now shows a connection between chronic stress, inflammation, and rising numbers of cardiovascular disease cases, and the research is revolutionizing how doctors treat cardiovascular disease. The American College of Cardiology is in agreement that the effects of acute and chronic stress on the sympathetic and parasympathetic nervous systems contribute to cardiovascular disease, with often fatal outcomes.[1]

Making things more problematic for first responders, current studies on work-related stress indicates that burnout is a risk factor for cardiovascular disease. Once again, the explanation seems to be chronic stress leading to an out-of-balance HPA axis.[2]

What affects the mind affects the heart, and vice versa

When I searched the PubMed database using the keywords "cardiovascular disease" and "depression," I got results from over 35 thousand studies. This is indisputably a hot topic!

Research is connecting the dots to show that heart disease is a mind-body issue. For example, one 2018 study published in *Frontiers of Neuroimmunology* reports that low-grade chronic inflammation is associated with higher incidences of depression and that "chronic depression is now listed among the most important cardiovascular risk factors for poor prognosis among patients with myocardial infarction [heart attacks]."[3]

What does this mean for firefighters? Every time I walk into a conference or firehouse to do a wellness presentation, I get excited because I show up with loads of clinical evidence supporting the beneficial effects of yoga and meditation on cardiovascular disease. Johns Hopkins Medicine, for example, gives this terrific overview:

> **Does Meditation Really Reduce Stress?**
>
> A 2017 study in the *Journal of Psychiatric Research* is particularly significant because it not only looked at 45 studies of different types of meditation but also used control groups to validate if meditation really helps reduce the effects of stress. The researchers found that *meditation reduced cortisol, blood pressure, heart rate, triglycerides, and inflammation markers.*[5]

One of yoga's clearest benefits to the heart is its ability to relax the body and mind. Emotional stress can cause a cascade of physical effects, including the release of hormones like cortisol and adrenaline, which narrow your arteries and increase blood pressure. The deep breathing and mental focus of yoga can offset this stress. Beyond off-loading stress, practicing yoga may help lower blood pressure, blood cholesterol, and blood glucose levels, as well as heart rate, making it a useful lifestyle intervention. Another study has shown that slow-paced yoga classes twice a week reduced the frequency of atrial fibrillation episodes in patients with that condition. In another report, patients with heart failure who went through an eight-week yoga program showed improvement in exercise capacity and quality of life. They also had lower blood levels of markers for inflammation, which contributes to heart disease.[4]

Heart rate variability shows your resiliency

We all know about the importance of a healthy heart rate, and athletes and first responders keep close track of their numbers because changes can signal problems. However, *heart rate variability* (HRV) is a newer marker for determining how balanced our autonomic nervous system is—and thus how resilient we are to stress, both physical and psychological.

While heart rate measures the average heartbeats per minute, HRV measures the variability between each heartbeat. In other words, how much the length of time between each heartbeat changes. Here's how it works: when you're under stress or exercising, on the one hand, your heart beats faster to get your blood pressure up and produce the extra oxygen you need. Both inhalation and exhalation phases are short and look very similar in length on the HRV readout. When there's very little variation, your HRV is low. When you're relaxed, on the other hand, your heart rate slows down on the exhalation phase, so the HRV readout shows shorter and then longer intervals between beats. You show a lot more variability—thus a high HRV.

If your HRV is still low even while you're in a resting or nonactive mode, that indicates that your fight-or-flight response is not shutting down. Not surprisingly, this is a common reading in people with traumatic stress. More than 20 years of research shows a relationship between low HRV and depression, anxiety, and cardiovascular disease.[6]

Resiliency—and how well your vagus nerve is doing its job

What HRV is really measuring is how well your vagus nerve is doing its job. Good *vagal tone*, as the scientists call it, means you're efficiently sending messages back and forth to the brain to manage your stress load (if this doesn't make sense, refer back to the "Parasympathetic Nervous System" section of chapter 4). The better your vagal tone, the faster you can switch gears from sympathetic to parasympathetic, and the more resilient you are, physically and mentally. Who would have thought that resiliency is really just another word for vagal tone!

Of course, I'm simplifying explanations of highly complex processes. Still, if you need another reason to add yoga to your daily routine, here it is: yoga, meditation, biofeedback, and breathing all have been shown to stimulate the vagal nerve, reduce inflammation, and improve HRV.[7]

How can you measure your HRV to make sure your yoga routine is working? We used to have to go to the doctor's office and have our electrocardiogram analyzed, but easy-to-use computer software and smartphone apps are now available to track your HRV. Using an app, you can check your HRV in the morning after you wake up, when it should be high. Then use it during the day to determine how well you recover from a stressful incident.

Depression, Anxiety, and PTSD

What happens when your job requires more than you can endure? This is a question I find myself asking a lot more often as I see how stress is affecting the first responders I work with.

I just read a first-of-its-kind mental health survey of 4,900 police, firefighters, and 911 call dispatchers in Fairfax County, VA, published in 2019. Fairfax County is heavily populated and represents the kinds of urban stressors first responders across the country face. The findings were stark: respondents had suicidal thoughts at a rate more than double the general population. Almost a quarter reported work-related depression, and nearly half couldn't stop looking for threats even in their own homes, a common symptom in people who have been exposed to trauma.[8]

First responders are well aware there's a problem, yet I've found that many don't have a clear understanding of just how profoundly chronic stress can decrease their mental resilience to the demands of the job. The prevailing warrior culture is certainly a powerful factor. In the survey, 30% of the first responders feared getting help because of the stigma around behavioral health issues. Part of the masculine mythology is that feeling or showing emotions are signs of weakness, and any sign of weakness can be deeply uncomfortable to someone who is tasked with saving others. First responders pride themselves on being a tight-knit society working together in dangerous environments and relying on each other for survival. Individuals with that preference for action may be unwilling or unable to step out of their comfort zone and ask, "What's going on with you?" when a colleague withdraws or fails to respond to questions or concerns.

No single person experiences life the same way as another, and depression and anxiety affect people differently for many different reasons. Looking at the many factors that influence behavioral health is outside the scope of this book, and I have kept the focus on the role of chronic stress on behavioral health issues and how yoga and meditation can help you do something about it. Overwhelmingly, hundreds of studies on yoga and meditation have found evidence that yoga can improve symptoms of depression, anxiety, stress, and PTSD and support life satisfaction and happiness. This section shares some of the best research on how it works.

The cytokine storm—the HPA axis, cortisol, and inflammation

Not surprisingly, given what we know about chronic stress, researchers are identifying an HPA axis in overdrive and producing high levels of cortisol as a significant factor in some people suffering from depression and anxiety.[9] Where there is high cortisol, inflammation often follows, with cytokines playing a major role.

Cytokines, those prolific and mysterious proteins I mentioned in the introduction to this chapter, are made by the immune system. Cytokines act as chemical messengers to our cells, and are rapidly becoming one of the hot topics for neuroscientists because they go pretty much everywhere in the body and affect everything from how we think to how we feel. For example, certain cytokines access parts of the brain where they activate key neurotransmitters that regulate our emotions, including *serotonin*, which affects anxiety, happiness, and mood; *dopamine*, which affects motivation and cognition; and *norepinephrine*, which affects alertness, energy, and memory.[10]

What happens when the HPA axis is in overdrive? Research suggests that signals go out to the immune system to produce too many pro-inflammatory cytokines, which can end up suppressing the immune system. The more researchers learn, the more robust is the connection to behavioral health. Some patients suffering from depression, for example, have been found to have higher levels of pro-inflammatory cytokines. Just how severe anxiety might become is also linked to certain cytokines.[11] Some early studies have indicated that these inflammatory cytokines may be associated with depressed patients who have attempted suicide.[12]

Cytokines affect your breathing

It's time to circle back to the breath. There's a reason many of the stories in this book are from firefighters who have found the breathing exercises in yoga and mindfulness to be life changing.

Cytokines transmit most of their messages via the vagus nerve, and yoga and meditation, with their ability to stimulate the vagus nerve through the breath, help the nervous system to reduce inflammatory cytokines and improve resilience.[13] Harvard Health recently reported that study participants in a three-month yoga and meditation retreat showed more protective cytokines and fewer harmful pro-inflammatory cytokines. They felt less depressed and anxious, and had fewer physical symptoms.[14] Remember, the very long vagus nerve runs directly through the digestive tract.

Start listening to your gut-brain connection

Pretty much everyone in the medical establishment is now telling us to listen to our gut-brain connection. Best-selling authors Justin Sonnenburg and Erica Sonnenburg call it the "good gut." So why should you start listening? Because this is an information super-highway that has a key role in balancing stress and emotions and that researchers are increasingly looking toward in connection with PTSD.[15]

The gut and brain communicate with each other through, you guessed it, the vagus nerve, sending continuous messages about the state of the mind–body. Thus, when you feel butterflies in your stomach or have that sinking feeling that happens when you head out on certain calls, you're getting messages from your gut that you're stressed. It seems the digestive system is particularly sensitive to emotional or psychological stress, a fact anyone with gastrointestinal sensitivity knows firsthand.

Neuroscientists now think the gut–brain communication could help fear management and PTSD through regulating signals coming from the gut to the amygdala, the part of the brain regulating fear and cognition. A groundbreaking study in the *Journal of Neuroscience* suggested that stimulating the vagus nerve "might be able to speed up the process by which people with PTSD can learn to reassociate a non-threatening stimuli which triggers anxiety with a neutral and non-traumatic experience."[16] This sounds much like the ability to let go of negative judgments that we get from practicing mindfulness!

Over the years, a number of studies have shown that people who practice mindfulness are more resilient to symptoms of PTSD. In one study, 117 veterans with PTSD who practiced mindfulness for eight weeks had significantly reduced symptoms.[17] The two facets of mindfulness practices identified as most helpful in reducing the severity of PTSD symptoms, including suicide risk, were *acting with awareness*, which means noticing what's happening in the moment, and *nonjudging inner experiences*, which means recognizing that a thought is just a thought.

A 2019 mindfulness study with 831 urban career firefighters is of particular interest because it builds on previous research implicating shame and guilt with PTSD and suicide risk. The study team found that firefighters who were able to "not judge themselves for having those feelings and instead might view the shame and guilt as an understandable response to their circumstances" were less at risk for suicidal thoughts and behaviors.[18]

In traditional warrior culture, shame and guilt are completely opposite of ideal: a person (typically a man) who is always brave, always doing the right thing, while conquering fear and doing whatever is necessary to get the job done. Sounds wonderful, like in television shows from 1950s all the way to *Chicago Fire* or *9-1-1*. However, this is not the reality I know from growing up in a fire family and from my work with first responders.

The emerging evidence that mind-body approaches can be effective at reducing PTSD symptoms is especially exciting because traditional interventions such as medication and psychotherapy, while beneficial for many people, have remission rates of only 20%–30% with combat veterans.[19] Scientist Akshya Vasudev is conducting a major year-long study in Canada on how yoga and meditation can be used to manage posttraumatic stress in first responders. In Vasudev's initial pilot study, first responders showed significant improvement in PTSD symptoms after practicing yoga for 12 weeks and even better results at week 24. As he puts it, "It's time to look at other ways to address the issue."[20]

Sleep Problems

Most firefighters I talk to struggle with sleep issues, particularly after long shifts or highly emotional calls. The problem quickly drifts into a chronic feedback loop: not enough sleep contributes to stress, and this stress then makes it harder to sleep. A study of 7,000 firefighters found that more than 37% suffered from sleep disorders.[21] For first responders, this can be deadly.

One yoga teacher shared with me her tragic motivation for seeking certification through my fire station yoga program. Her son, who had been a volunteer firefighter for a short time and loved his job, loved helping people, fell asleep at the wheel after finishing a long shift and was killed. She told me the outpouring of support from his department for her and her family was so moving and heartfelt that she wanted to honor her son and give back to his "other family" by giving them some tools to better manage the demands of the job.

Sleep issues affect your health

The costs of not sleeping are all encompassing. According to Harvard Health, "Sleep disruption—which affects levels of neurotransmitters and stress hormones, among other things—wreaks havoc in the brain, impairing thinking and emotional regulation."[22] In addition, sleep disruption imparts higher risks for other conditions. In one article that looked at a number of epidemiological studies, the authors concluded that not sleeping enough is associated with "increased incidence of cardiovascular diseases, such as coronary artery disease, hypertension, arrhythmias, diabetes, and obesity."[23]

Although a number of factors contribute to sleep problems, an overactive HPA axis is one of the top culprits. Cortisol is the hormone responsible for regulating sleep cycles, so it's believable that overly high levels of this stress hormone might disrupt sleep.[24] First responders, like professional athletes, typically have a lot of adrenaline and cortisol in

Better Sleep

Here's an easy tip that any firehouse can use to promote better sleep (check out Toomey's website Firstrespondersleeprecovery.com for more strategies):

> The circadian rhythm is dictated by exposure to light and dark, and blue light exposure causes the production of cortisol, which suppresses melatonin. So having red light bulbs or low spectrum blue bulbs in sleeping areas are easy ways to promote better rest.

—Jacqueline Toomey, First Responder Sleep Recovery Program

their bodies because the job demands peak performance, making winding down at the end of a shift particularly challenging.

So the big idea here is that it's critically important to do something about any sleep problems you might have. One of the simplest, most effective ways to get to sleep is using yoga and meditation to calm down the stress response system. I commonly hear firefighters reporting that they experience their best night of sleep following one of our classes in the station.

An article in the *Journal of the American Medical Association* found that participants in a clinical trial measuring the effectiveness of mindfulness meditation on sleep disorders had less insomnia, fatigue, and depression at the end of only six sessions.[25] In a study published in the journal *Sleep*, a mindfulness-based stress reduction program, particularly one designed for sleep disorders, significantly reduced the severity of insomnia for chronic sufferers. What I find most encouraging in the study is that the difference was largest at the three-month follow-up—results that last![26]

I had an inspiring conversation with Jacqueline Toomey, founder and director of the First Responder Sleep Recovery Program in Denver. A lifelong practitioner of yoga and meditation, Toomey realized the healing power of her practice when it facilitated her recovery from a traumatic brain and spinal cord injury after a car accident. Then she married a firefighter and found out how much trauma they experience on the job, especially when her husband lost a senior partner to suicide. Toomey decided to create a yoga program that focused specifically on sleep issues for first responders, incorporating the best information on neurochemistry. "All the research in the last 10–15 years proved what the ancient wisdom of yoga has always known," Toomey told me. "When you manipulate the body in certain ways and control the breath, it will ultimately shift the nervous system. The parasympathetic nervous system calms body and mind to promote healing, and neurotransmitters in the brain are released, particularly serotonin, a precursor to melatonin, the sleep hormone."

Cancer and sleep

The relationship between sleep and cancer is also being studied. The sleep research that Toomey discussed is pertinent for firefighters because it shows the negative impact of shift work on our *circadian rhythm*—the sleep–wake cycle that is critical to our ability to sleep well. The International Agency for Research on Cancer in a 2019 review of the research suggested that circadian rhythm disruption, which leads to low melatonin levels, is "probably carcinogenic to humans."[27]

With more research being conducted on the impact of sleep, scientists are hypothesizing that during sleep is when our bodies repair any DNA damage to our neurons. Melatonin is a key player because it regulates this sleep–wake cycle. When the cycle is disrupted, whether by shift work or other stress that causes our circadian rhythm to go haywire, our cells can be more susceptible to cancer-causing mutations.[28] On the positive side, studies that are using melatonin along with chemotherapy are finding that melatonin "increases survival time and reduces the toxic side effects from chemotherapy."[29]

Chronic Pain

I was shocked when I read in the *Washington Post* that "the many varieties of chronic pain make up the most common and disabling health problem in the world." This statement makes more sense when you learn that medical professionals actually know very little about how to deal with pain. Benjamin Kligler, national director of the Integrative Health Coordinating Center at the Veterans Health Administration, says this is because pain is so complex and "interwoven with all kinds of psychological, emotional, and spiritual dimensions, as well as the physical."[30]

We do know that attention, fatigue, distraction, mood, and emotions like fear and anger are factors in how we experience pain and determine whether our pain will become chronic. Genetics also plays a role, and some of us are more susceptible to feeling pain or feeling it more intensely. What's extremely frustrating to those of us who practice mind–body approaches to wellness is that stress is rarely considered in pain rehabilitation.[31] This seems to fly in the face of all we're learning about the role of cortisol in producing excess inflammation in the body and about inflammation's role as a major cause of pain. Furthermore, stress plays a role in activating the fear and avoidance parts of the brain, which significantly affects our response to pain.

I love this quote from the journal *Physical Therapy*: "Stress may be unavoidable in life, and challenges are inherent to success; however, humans have the capability to modify what they perceive as stressful and how they respond to it."[32] This is exactly the principle behind how yoga and meditation work and why the U.S. Armed Services are so interested in them (see chapter 2). When you're on the mat, you're not only calming the stress response system and lowering inflammation, but also practicing the kind of awareness and attention that builds your ability to regulate your responses, develop a more flexible mindset, and have more control over how to handle chronic pain. Some of the most rewarding conversations I've had with firefighters have been when they started talking about their pain not with resignation, but with hope.

Self-Regulation: Transforming Chronic Stress into Good Stress

One of the most common occurrences at the end of a yoga class is that firefighters leave happier than when they started. Maybe they're smiling, cracking jokes, or just looking "lighter" than they did an hour earlier. A big part of what's happening is that yoga is helping them transform their chronic stress into good stress by strengthening their ability to self-regulate.

Self-regulation is how we control our behavior and emotions to achieve our long-term goals. Self-regulation is the key to resilience. When you can calm yourself down when upset and shift your mood from negative to optimistic, you're better able to keep a more flexible mindset and maintain the motivation you need to pursue your dreams.

In one of my favorite investigations into how yoga works, top researchers looked at hundreds of studies to see if self-regulation was indeed a factor for success. The researchers linked classical components of yoga to modern, scientific concepts using the following four components:

- Ethical principles
- Sustained poses
- Breath regulation
- Meditation techniques

Calling yoga "meditation in action," these researchers looked at how the practice affected each part of the brain, from the autonomic nervous system to other parts of the brain that are responsible for fear and how we make decisions and create our worldview.[33] Here's my summary of their key finding: while you're on the mat during yoga class, you're practicing *intentional concentration*—focusing on particular sensations to the exclusion of others.

This kind of focused attention that happens while you're doing the poses, breathing, and mindfulness exercises creates *cognitive flexibility*. This capacity in turn will help you to focus on what's important in any situation and disregard what's not important. Therefore, rather than being on autopilot, you're better able to let go of habitual responses or negative emotions, for example, that might interfere with your judgment. The heavy backpack that you might be carrying around is lighter, giving you more mental bandwidth for making decisions. Furthermore, because your autonomic nervous system is more in balance, you're able to put on the brakes more quickly after an emergency.

When you put it all together, you're creating a feedback loop that reinforces positive responses. You're transforming your negative stress into good stress. You're building your resilience. When firefighters come back from a call and tell me they reacted more calmly, with greater patience and equanimity than usual, self-regulation is one of the main reasons.

Conclusion

The firefighters participating in yoga programs know they can email me with questions or comments any time. It's one of the ways I keep in touch with what's happening because some stations are so busy there isn't a lot of time for conversation before or after classes. I recently got an email from "Greg," a career firefighter in his fifties who had never tried yoga before. I wasn't sure what Greg thought about the classes because he didn't say much at the time. But when he reached out via email, he let me know he was feeling much more flexible and energetic afterward. The biggest change for him, though, was connected to mental stress and anxiety. He said that after his second class, the stress he used to feel was gone—and not only at work, but at home, too. Before he goes to sleep at night, he goes into the Savasana pose and uses the breathing exercises he practiced during classes.

This is not to say all first responders will react the same. Stress is a huge topic, with enormous impact. It's like a complex stew, made up of all the stressors that affect our inner and outer worlds: genetics, early life experiences, where we live, our jobs, personal relationships, and all those emotions that add extra spice and flavor (sometimes too much). Yoga and meditation work by giving you a way to experience your relationship with these stressors differently. Simply by being present in the moment and practicing nonjudgment, you trigger your mind–body system to start doing what it has evolved to do—regulate stress and return the body to homeostasis. It's a very different experience from the way most of us live our lives.

In the next chapter, you'll learn the nuts and bolts of how FireFlex Yoga is designed specifically to help firefighters transform their relationship with stress and how you can incorporate the principles into your department. In later chapters, I will explain how particular yoga poses and mindfulness meditations can change your brain and enable you to cultivate essential competencies like functional fitness, situational awareness, decision-making, emotional intelligence, and overall fulfillment and well-being.

Part IV

How to Set Up an Evidence-Based Yoga Program in Your Fire Station

6

Fireflex Yoga Fundamentals
EVERYTHING YOU NEED TO KNOW

Know Your Audience

I have spent months studying what firefighters do, analyzing their every movement and poring over injury reports to identify the most common injuries. I had endless conversations with my father and firefighter friends to find ways to make the program practical geared to the needs firefighters have for performing intensively and staying healthy throughout their careers. But nothing prepared me for actually hearing the stories as firefighters returned to yoga class after a call.

Quickly, I saw that vastly different calls require different kinds of preparation, both operationally and tactically, for which mind–body integration could lay the foundation. It was surprising to me how little mental conditioning there was for helping first responders not just to cope with what they see every day but to ground themselves amid chaos and situations that are sometimes full of huge adrenaline spikes and other times boring and mundane.

All career firefighters have access to behavioral health assistance through their *employee assistance program* (EAP). But I'm also aware that firefighters tend to give their EAPs poor reviews. As all the reports point out, the stigma of getting help and the perception (many times accurately) that counselors don't understand first responder culture keep many firefighters from reaching out. The NFPA's Center for Excellence was created to promote better behavioral health and mental resilience; however, as with counseling, their programs are based on talking as the primary means of delivery, and the demand for services far exceed their capacity to meet those demands. Moreover, we know how the warrior culture views talking about emotions and feelings, especially being vulnerable, as signs of weakness unworthy of a proud tradition.

One beauty of yoga is that you don't have to talk—especially about your feelings! In fact, firefighters often tell me that yoga class is the first time they've ever been in a room full of firefighters where the room was quiet and peaceful because no one was posturing and making wisecracks.

This chapter will give you the fundamental components of how to bring a program like this to your department as well as results from data collection over four years. Essential concepts like functional movement are often misunderstood or underutilized. My conversations with Josh LaRoe, engineer and American Council on Exercise (ACE)-certified peer fitness trainer at the Vacaville Fire Department in California, zero in on exactly why functional movement should be part of any successful yoga program. While every department has its unique culture, the general guidelines presented here can be adapted to the priorities of any department.

Building Mind-Body Resilience

Objectives

The following four objectives form the core of this program and have been refined on the basis of the results of more than 1,000 firefighters who have completed the program:

- Increasing movement awareness
- Reducing the rate and severity of injuries
- Lessening the negative effects of chronic and traumatic stress, particularly by increasing interoception
- Developing cognitive flexibility, open mindset, and mental conditioning to create more effective leadership

Location

Classes are typically 60 minutes long and are held at the fire station during physical training time. The most common locations for classes are in the dayroom for smaller class sizes or in the apparatus bay, union hall, conference room, or training facility for multiple engine companies.

Measurement

To customize yoga classes and to measure results after the program is completed, FireFlex Yoga uses pre- and postprogram assessments: the *Functional Movement Screen* (FMS) and a body awareness screen called the *Multidimensional Assessment of Interoceptive Awareness* (MAIA). Before you integrate the FMS into your station's fitness program, it's important to understand functional fitness.

Functional Fitness: Identifying Who Is at Risk for Injury

Joint mobility and muscle flexibility can affect firefighters' range of motion and either inhibit or enhance safety and performance. My yoga program starts with where to get the most bang for the buck: strains and sprains. These are not only the most common injuries reported by firefighters but also the most costly. A fitness program can help by focusing on learning how to move well and how to move often. Yoga's focus on body awareness is the foundation of any good functional movement program!

Functional movement isn't a new concept in the fire service. But at the individual station level, many firefighters don't fully understand what it is and how improving the way they move can help them to avoid injuries or to speed up their recovery time when they do unavoidably get injured.

Functional fitness is about patterns

Functional fitness isn't strength training. It's not traditional fitness training that works on isolated parts of the body. It looks at movement patterns instead. Think of it this way: when you squat down to pick up a patient on a gurney or pick up your child, you're basically doing the same thing: using the same set of muscles and the same movement patterns. If these are movements you do all the time, you can become habituated to performing the movement incorrectly, and the likelihood of sustaining an injury increases. When you scrutinize these movement patterns, imbalances and limited range of motion can be discovered, and you gain the knowledge to do something about it.[1] It's a systems approach: if one part is not working properly, then that part will affect the whole.

Movement awareness starts at the academy

Strength and conditioning functional fitness practices similar to CrossFit are becoming more prevalent in fire academies today, which are effective at providing a broad spectrum of training modalities to athletes. When I talked to Josh LaRoe about his experience as a trainer for the Vacaville, CA, Fire Department, he told me that functional fitness is an extremely effective training protocol. "Having a well-rounded fitness plan and being physically fit and able to perform a task are key abilities in the fire service," he said. "But being physically fit isn't everything. It's equally important that firefighters stay conditioned to move properly because many injuries occur due to lack of proper movement fundamentals and flexible mobility."

I asked LaRoe about the recruits he trains at the academy and his assessment of their movement patterns. "Even in 16 weeks," he said, "I could never get some recruits to properly execute a barbell dead lift from the ground without compromising their lower backs due to hip immobility—even when I added mobility and flexibility exercises daily throughout the 16 weeks." He explained that he would have to make accommodations, such as starting the lift a few inches higher from the ground so the hips would slowly open up enough and allow the lumbar spine to maintain a neutral position.

What can this kind of immobility lead to? LaRoe explained, "Everything we do in the fire service is lifting heavy stuff all day long. So firefighters have the potential to damage their bodies over time if they don't move properly."

What about physical abilities tests?

If you want to be a firefighter in California, you have to pass the Candidate Physical Ability Test (CPAT). It's the recognized standard for measuring an individual's ability to handle the physical demands of being a firefighter and covers many of the high-risk movements a firefighter needs to successfully perform on the job. The point is that just passing the test doesn't mean you're doing each of the movements in the safest, most efficient way, and over a long career, this can be problematic.

For a lot of the chronic pain that firefighters deal with, it's often impossible to remember a specific triggering incident. This is because rather than a single event, the problem results from repeating the same movement with poor form over and over. Hence what might not be a big problem in the short term can seriously affect you in the long run.

According to LaRoe, the CPAT is a decent enough predictor of whether a recruit can handle a physical load. Still, based on his training experience, he explained that "it doesn't necessarily discriminate for good or bad form, so someone can be violating several key movement features and still pass with a 100%. This is why ongoing education and practice in movement patterns is so important."

For example, the CPAT includes an equipment-carry test that functionally represents a potential movement on the fireground: lifting tools from shelf to ground, then picking the equipment back off the ground and carrying it from point A to point B. Now let's take this movement out to the field where firefighters respond to many daily emergencies. Let's say grabbing a heart monitor, medical bag, or other equipment weighing 20–60 pounds from one of the apparatus compartments. The equipment will probably be close to eye level or considerably above—not on the ground.

According to LaRoe, many firefighters take it for granted that they can just grab the equipment with one arm fully extended and pull it out. This equipment might be relatively lightweight, so what's the problem? The problem is that if you repeatedly load the shoulder in an internally rotated position, over time you can cause repeated trauma to your shoulder joint (for more on the shoulder, see chapter 9). By contrast, when firefighters learn to perform this movement pattern with awareness, they lift and pull the equipment close to their chest and grab it with two hands.

This point is so important because as LaRoe pointed out, roughly 70% of all emergencies firefighters respond to are medical, thereby constituting a considerable source of injuries in the fire service. LaRoe validated what I've seen in my work with the FMS when he explained that medical emergencies don't necessarily require more strength or stamina, as much as they draw on finesse and conscious or mindful movement patterns that don't violate the key features that would injure someone. This, in his opinion, "is the most difficult challenge universally for all tactical/industrial athletes, regardless of their daily occupation. To retrain the brain to have a conscious mind–body connection to maintain proper movement patterns takes a lot of time and effort."

If it takes know-how and discipline to move properly rather than conveniently or habitually, is it really worth it? After years of training recruits and going on calls, LaRoe summed up the answer this way: "Everything we do in our strength and conditioning training increases our threshold of what we can physically manage on an emergency incident without getting injured. If I stay physically fit and condition my movement patterns to be uncompromising, my risk of being injured during daily work is drastically reduced."

The Functional Movement Screen

The FMS (fig. 6–1) assesses seven unique movement patterns for mobility and stability (starting in the top left of the image and proceeding clockwise):

- Hurdle step
- Deep squat
- Shoulder mobility
- In-line lunge
- Trunk stability
- Rotary stability
- Active straight-leg raise

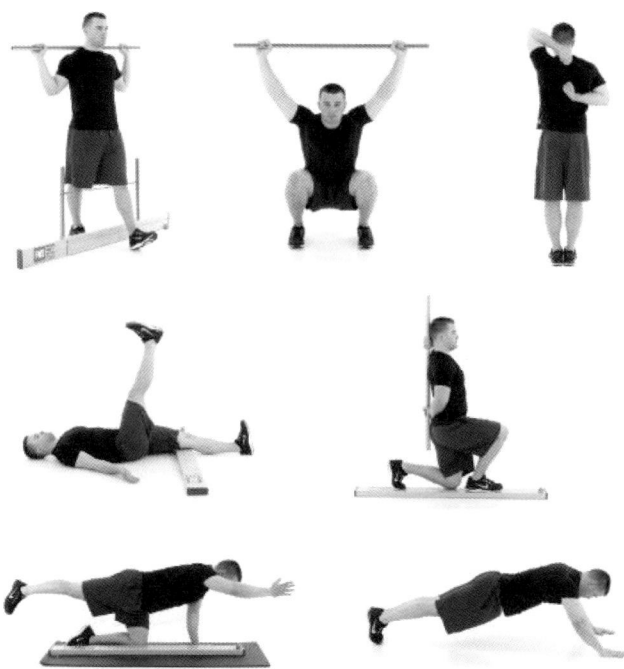

Figure 6-1.
Functional Movement Screen (FMS)

The idea of the FMS is that once you know how to move safely, you can work on strength and conditioning safely.[2] Note that the FMS is not a test; rather, it's a way to identify movement deficiencies that might put you or someone else at risk of injury.

In chapter 4, I talked about the yin-yang balance of homeostasis that we need to maintain for good health. The same principle applies here for physical resilience. It's harder for your body to bounce back after a strenuous call if some parts are too overtaxed to compensate for movement weaknesses. This is why the FMS is being used by the U.S. military and many professional sports teams. Being *fit for duty* is the most basic requirement for every firefighter, and performance depends directly on the ability to move safely, effectively, and routinely through fundamental movement patterns.

Economic impact and the FMS

Here's some excellent news from the Denver Fire Department. They have saved more than $8 million in workers' compensation claims since their new health and wellness program started in 2016. In the first year alone, the total cost for treating these injuries dropped 42%.[3] How are they getting these results? First, Denver's new health and wellness program, which covers physical and behavioral health, treats firefighters like professional athletes, which includes physical therapy every day as part of the rehabilitation process. Then there's a priority on movement education, with the FMS playing a key role.

Casey Stoneberger, director of physical therapy at the Denver Fire Department, and team have been embedded in the department for five years, going on ride-alongs, learning the fire culture, and gaining the trust of the firefighters. He said that they use the FMS before and after academies, "which gives common language everyone can understand.

Our records show an average of just under 2% increases in scores per academy class." After the success of the FMS in the fire academies, strength and conditioning trainers started using the FMS. Then the Denver Fire Department started using the FMS to discharge worker compensation claims for return to full duty. Stoneberger said this involved educating "everyone who was on work comp that they would have to pass the FMS again for their specific injury." This is a brilliant strategy because it means injured firefighters will pay more attention to a functional movement approach to rehabilitation, reducing the probability of reinjury.

How have firefighters responded to the FMS? Stoneberger said that in 2017 the department switched its voluntary fitness evaluation, which had a participation rate of 30%, to one that involved using a treadmill test and taking the FMS. What happened? Participation skyrocketed to almost 70%. Stoneberger credits the extensive education on the FMS and the successful outcomes from the program. It's hard to argue with success.

The good news that firefighters can improve their FMS scores is spreading to other fire departments. In a 2017 study, 55 active-duty firefighters increased their scores after an eight-week program.[4] Invariably, injuries will still happen. As Denver modeled, the FMS can act as a return-to-work standard that firefighters need to pass to demonstrate they truly are physically ready to go back. What a great idea, because many of the departments my yoga program works with don't yet have a return-to-work assessment.

Yoga and the FMS

I have created a graphic to show how closely the FMS tracks what firefighters do. Figure 6–2 shows common firefighter movements matched with those in the standard FMS.

Before they ever take a yoga class in my program, every firefighter participant takes the FMS. Their instructor then uses the overall results of the assessments to create a baseline for developing a sequence of classes. On the basis of these data, here's the sequence of the first 10 classes, which are paired according to five themes that cover the most common movement deficiencies:

- *Theme 1—hips.* Classes 1 and 2 develop hip mobility.
- *Theme 2—shoulders.* Classes 3 and 4 increase shoulder mobility.
- *Theme 3—trunk stability.* Classes 5 and 6 develop stability in the lumbar-pelvic complex and thoracic spine.
- *Theme 4—balance.* With appropriate mobility and stability in the hips, shoulders, and trunk, classes 7 and 8 incorporate asymmetric and single-leg balancing.
- *Theme 5—integration.* Classes 9 and 10 focus on balancing effort and ease and mobility and stability while moving (flowing) from pose to pose.

The results from more than four years of classes show that the FireFlex Yoga approach is improving functional fitness. My brilliant colleague Sonia Rackelmann, a researcher and certified FMS screener, crunched the data from four years of data from FireFlex Yoga programs. That consisted of pre- and postprogram FMS and MAIA assessments across seven departments from 2016 to 2019.

Figure 6–3 gives the data from the FMS scores. Seventy-six firefighters were assessed. Their overall FMS scores for six of the seven movement patterns show a decrease in scores of 0 or 1 and an increase in scores of 2 or 3. This means a decrease in pain or compensation in doing the movements, and an increase in more normal and acceptable levels of

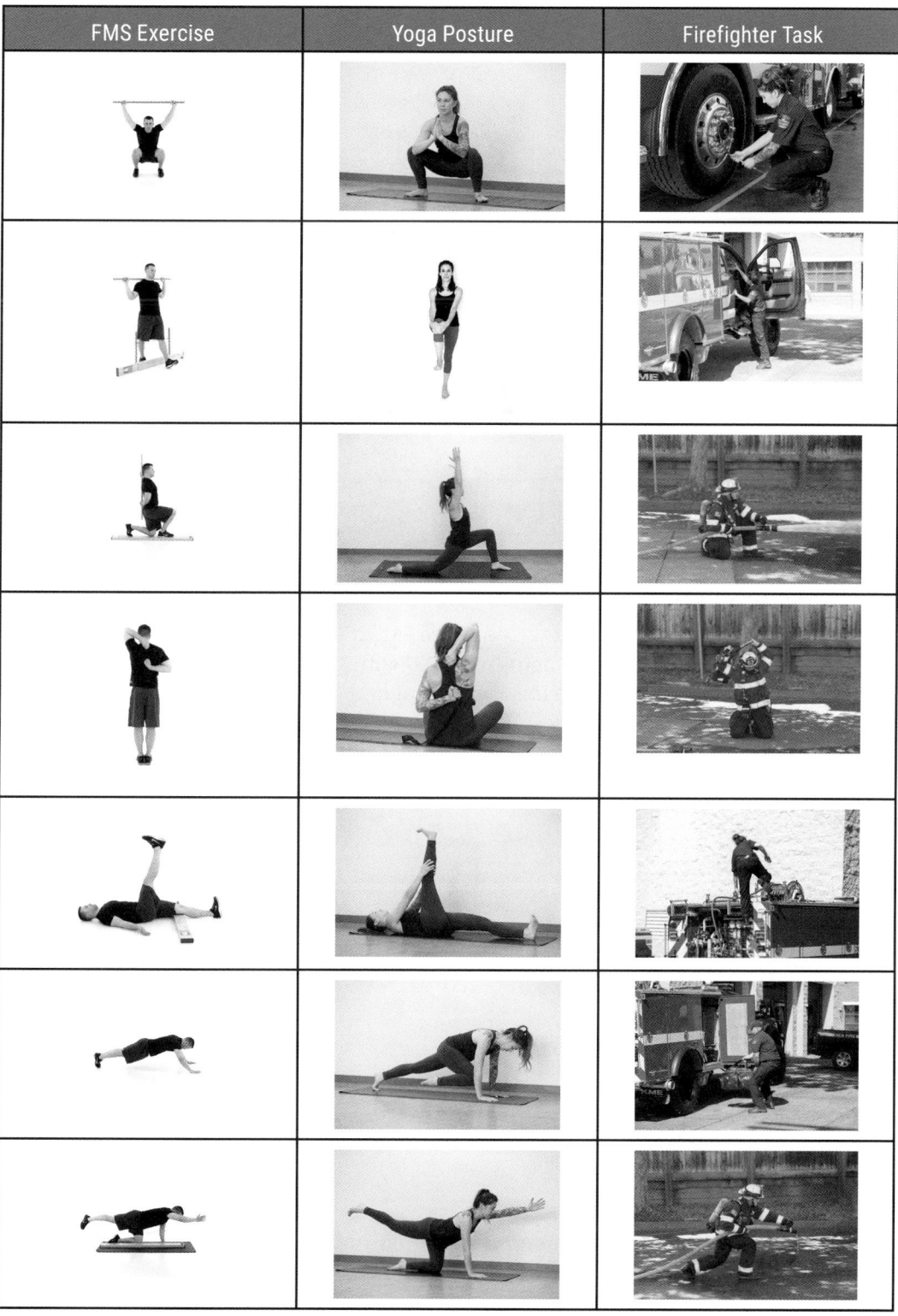

FMS Exercise	Yoga Posture	Firefighter Task

Figure 6-2.
FMS tracked over firefighter job tasks and yoga poses

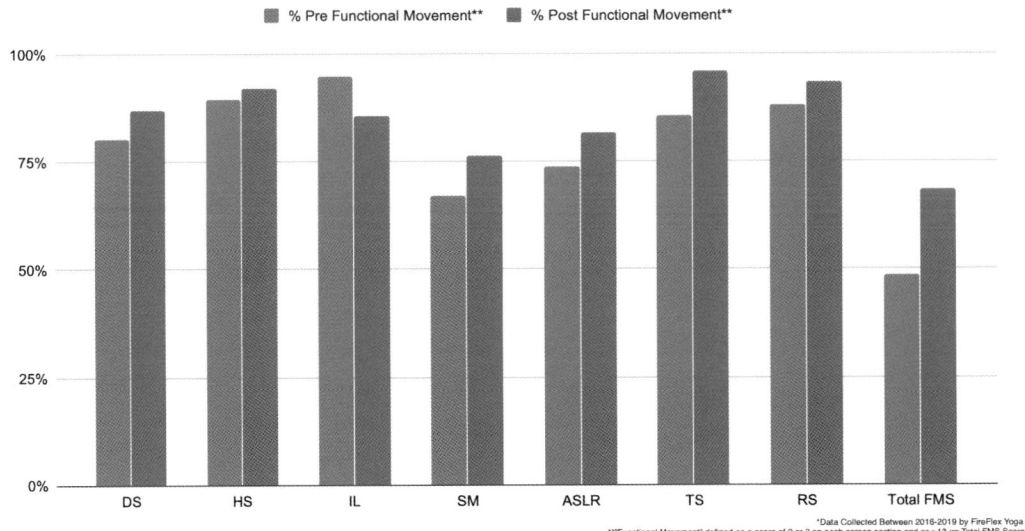

Figure 6–3.
Firefighters' FMS scores before and after yoga program (**N** = 76)
Note: DS = deep squat, HS = hurdle step, IL = inline lunge, SM = shoulder mobility, ASLR = active straight leg raise, TS = trunk stability, RS = rotary stability

compensation or no compensation at all needed. The only movement pattern that didn't show improvement was the in-line lunge. This is not surprising, since the first FireFlex Yoga program is only 10 sessions and focuses primarily on mobility and joint stability in the simpler movement patterns. We need more data on an extended program that would go for another 10 sessions to determine improvement in the in-line lunge.

The Multidimensional Assessment of Interoceptive Awareness

Optimal performance and overall well-being come from a combination of both physical and mental health. That's why the second measurement tool of the FireFlex Yoga program is the Multidimensional Assessment of Interoceptive Awareness (MAIA). This is a questionnaire that looks at how in tune someone is to what's happening in their body and how well they are managing that input. It's the most widely used self-reporting measure of interoceptive bodily awareness and has been translated into 40 languages. Chapter 3 explained what interoception is, but in this chapter, you'll learn how measuring it is critical for first responders.

A study that looked at 160 Olympic athletes found that a significant number of them did not perform up to their potential "because they were not prepared for the distractions they faced." In fact, researchers found the two most important skills affecting high performance levels were attentional focus and the quality of performance imagery. Other elements included total commitment to excellence, quality training, daily goal setting, quality of practice, quality mental preparation, and internal imagery.[5] How many of these factors have to do with high-level cognitive abilities and mental resilience, not just physical strength and conditioning?

The originator of the MAIA, Wolf Mehling, is an integrative physician and core research faculty member at University of California San Francisco's Osher Center for Integrative Medicine, as well as professor in the Department of Family and Community Medicine. Dr. Mehling has said that while the screen doesn't measure performance, it can reveal the degree to which people can trust their bodies and switch from thinking to sensing. This information can give a good indication of the level of stress a person is experiencing and their level of self-regulation, such as the ability to deal with distractions, set goals, and manage emotions.[6] These are key competencies firefighters need as much as Olympic athletes.

Here are the body-sensing capabilities measured on the MAIA and how they relate to those observed in the most resilient firefighters:

- *MAIA body-sensing capabilities*—noticing, nondistracting, not worrying, attention regulation, emotional awareness, self-regulation, body listening
- *Firefighter capabilities*—situational awareness, emotional intelligence, body awareness, careful listening, self-regulation, decision-making, agency

Yoga and the MAIA

Like the FMS, the MAIA is given to every firefighter before and after completing the FireFlex Yoga program. These scores give us some direction about how well firefighters are in tune with what's going on in their bodies and how well they are regulating their physiology and managing that input. The chart in Figure 6–4 shows results from more than four years of data.

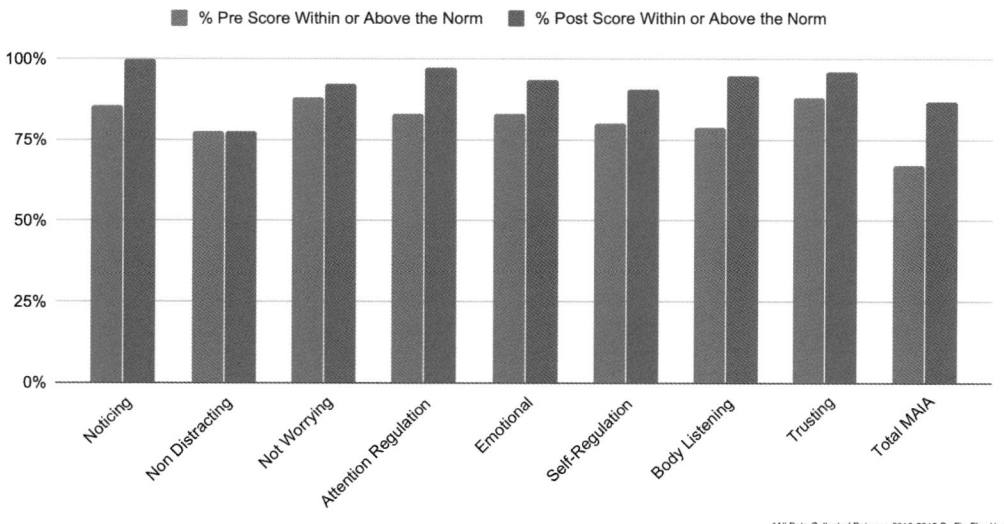

*All Data Collected Between 2016-2019 By FireFlex Yoga

Figure 6–4.
Percentage of pre- and post-MAIA scores compared to the norm in the general population (*N* = 76)

Seventy-six firefighters completed the MAIA. All firefighter scores that fell below one standard deviation of the mean were considered lower-range scores, while all scores that fell above one standard deviation of the mean were considered higher-range scores. A large majority of the firefighter population scored *within* this range, which in this case would be considered the normal range.

More interesting, though, is the change from before to after the program in terms of the percentage of firefighters who initially scored lower versus higher range. As Figure 6–4 shows, there was a general trend of more higher-range scores on individual scores, and especially noticeable was the change in total score before and after. Among other things, the scores suggest firefighters were self-regulating better, showing more awareness of their emotions, and were less distracted—all components of better decision-making and increased well-being. In other words, they achieved increased resilience.

The body keeps the score

In his groundbreaking and highly respected book on trauma, *The Body Keeps the Score*, neurobiologist Bessel van der Kolk expresses so eloquently why FireFlex Yoga uses the MAIA as a fundamental screening measurement:

> "Agency" is the technical term for the feeling of being in charge of your life, knowing where you stand, knowing that you have a say in what happens to you, knowing that you have some ability to shape your circumstances. . . . Agency starts with what scientists call interoception, our awareness of our subtle sensory, body-based feelings: the greater that awareness, the greater our potential to control our lives. Knowing what we feel is the first step to knowing why we feel that way. . . . This is why mindfulness practice, which strengthens the MPFC [medial prefrontal cortex of the brain] is a cornerstone of recovering from trauma.[7]

Neuroplasticity: A Bicep Curl to the Brain

How do we strengthen our brains to develop more agency, or increase our endurance and resilience, or change a dysfunctional movement pattern? Science calls the process *neuroplasticity*—the remarkable capacity of the brain to rewire itself to adapt to new information. The Cleveland Clinic explains that neuroplasticity "allows your brain to be jump-started, fine-tuned, and remodeled throughout your adult life."[8]

Forming pathways, or connections, is how the millions of neurons in our brain communicate with each other. Each neuron in a pathway talks to the other via electrical and chemical pulsations. New brains cells form, creating new pathways, and old circuits that we don't use get discarded. We can influence this process by consciously lighting up those connections through practice and repetition of new thoughts and actions. In other words, we should continue to exercise those pathways that we want to keep—hence the adage "use it or lose it." Thus, every time you engage in learning something new, whether a tactical procedure, another language, or a new yoga pose, your brain starts activating the neurons in the part of the brain responsible for learning and memory, and you start creating new neural circuits.[9] If you keep exercising these neurons, not only will you acquire new physical or mental strength, but you'll also be creating the long-term habit of learning.

Psychologist and best-selling author Rick Hanson has explained why neuroplasticity grants us such an open mindset and increased mental resilience. Dr. Hanson makes the analogy that the brain "is Teflon for good experiences and Velcro for bad."[10] What he means is that because of negativity bias (see chapter 3), especially when compounded by chronic stress, many of us have etched deep pathways in our brain that light up messages of unhappiness, disappointment, fatigue, or anxiety, and our brains tend to go down one of those pathways no matter what happens. We acknowledge these pathways as negative habits and beliefs. However, the same neuroplastic ability of the brain to create these negative pathways can be used to create more beneficial pathways to better habits and new beliefs. Abundant research now shows that yoga and meditation are particularly good at helping us rewire our brains to create more resilient pathways so we can move better, think better, and handle pain and stress better.[11]

Conclusion

Bringing yoga to the firehouse is not intended to convert CrossFit-loving firefighters into yogis. It's to make the case, "You love your job? You want to be at the firehouse working and not laid up on your couch binge-watching *Ozark*? Then try adding yoga and meditation into your daily routine." In the next six chapters, you can see the classes themselves as firefighters practice yoga and mindfulness and then take what they learn on the mat into their lives, at work and at home.

7

Day One

Lesson 1: This Ain't No Yoga Studio

Depending on where a fire station yoga class is being held—in the dayroom or apparatus bay—the first smells to greet me when I walk are either bacon, eggs, and coffee or engine exhaust, oil, and disinfectant. I prefer coffee and prefer when we practice in the dayroom. However, not all fire departments have a choice. Some departments have so much history or are so old that their dayrooms are barely large enough for a few recliners and a television set. The newly built fire departments, on the other hand, have fitness centers or dayrooms large enough to hold classes.

Then there's the noise. Because we deliver classes to on-duty firefighters, radio and dispatcher noise can interrupt the quiet at any time. Obviously, crews need to hear the dispatch, so there's no getting around this entirely. However, some crews—and certainly battalion chiefs—also like to hear calls coming in for neighboring stations, to get early alerts of potential larger incidents. There are advantages and disadvantages to having classes in such a noisy environment. Even though the noisy background is not ideal for beginners, experiencing yoga in our native environment will over time encourage integration, busting the myth that yoga happens only in some Zen space. Rather, yoga is the connection you feel each time you take a conscious breath wherever you are! Firefighters learn how to wind down the nervous system and find calm in the middle of the chaos.

Lesson 2: Don't Forget Your Yoga Socks

The first day of a 10-week program brings a lot of anticipation. The typical scenario runs something like this: the firefighters aren't sure what to expect, but they're fitted out with their physical training gear—department-issued shorts and T-shirts that are to be worn while working out—and the yoga mats have been laid out in neat rows. Practically everyone has their socks on. Some are even standing on their mats with their shoes on. That is until I tell them that their face is going to be on that mat. They quickly hop off, but are still reluctant to take off their socks.

After teaching in traditional yoga studios for years, this puzzled me until one day I asked and got this answer: "What type of respectable workout regime requires you to go barefoot?" Especially when your workspace might be filled with biohazardous materials tracked in on your boots! This is something my dad would have said, so I got it. And once I explain that bare feet give better traction and resistance on yoga mats for a better work-out, they get it. By the end of the 10 weeks many of the firefighters went from wearing CrossFit shoes, to socks, to yoga socks, which are good for yoga even where bare feet wouldn't be safe or acceptable.

In fact, teaching yoga in a firehouse is different in a number of ways. In a typical yoga studio, before class I would find students quietly doing warm-up stretches, meditating, or lying in Savasana pose for a discrete catnap. Definitely not standing on their mats, arms crossed, engaging in raucous conversations with the others. But what can I say? Firefighters have captured my heart. Camaraderie is what makes teaching inside a firehouse so special, and the expressions of gratitude are windows into what firefighters feel once their armor has come off. I'm teaching people who already interact like a family, who trust each other with their lives. And this is established long before day one.

Lesson 3: Yoga Begins When Someone Farts

Shortly after I started FireFlex Yoga, I hired a teacher who, adhering to the traditions of her yoga-teaching lineage, found the rowdy behavior at the beginning of many firehouse yoga classes unsettling. Not knowing what else to do, she told the firefighters to shush. Even though they did quiet down and settled into the routine of the class, the teacher lost credibility and shortly stopped teaching at that department. This was a wake-up call for me, and I quickly enhanced the section in my teacher certification course on understand-ing fire culture. I wanted my teachers to better understand the role of respect in bringing yoga and fire traditions together and that firefighters are most comfortable when they can joke and cajole with each other.

So now when I see shoes on, I know where it's coming from. I know the laughter and conversations are simply ways to discharge some of the discomfort or awkwardness about standing on a yoga mat next to your crew and rig, with your turns out set up just beyond the mat. I know everyone will start to quiet down, and I do say a few words at the begin-ning of the class to set expectations, discuss the focus of the class, and remind firefighters that in spite of their extremely busy schedule and the need to be doing six things at the same time, they have made an excellent choice to slow down for the next 60 minutes.

I remind them that this is exactly the rest and recharge they need in order to leave class and dive back into the fray of their lives with more energy and vigor. I explain that there is no doubt in my mind that in the beginning this choice comes with a certain amount of inner conflict, which is understandable. Yoga is different, it can be awkward, and it's perceived in our society as something done mainly by women. This last point is extremely important because of the prevalence of the male chauvinistic warrior culture in the fire service. On day one, I just touch on this idea, but I will gradually expand on it as the classes progress.

Class 1 Objective: Is Everybody Happy?

In all seriousness, my primary objective for class 1 is to make sure that everyone shows up for class 2. Not everyone is happy about having a yoga class inside their station. I've seen firefighters who intentionally disrupt class—by walking through the dayroom during class with their boots on and step all over the mats, or going into the kitchen adjacent to the dayroom and clattering baking pans, or blaring rock music in the neighboring gym while loudly dropping weights on the floor. When something like this happens, it's challenging to keep the group on the mats from feeling angry or unsupported. Initially, I was surprised how rarely the person making a ruckus was asked to quiet down. I am fairly comfortable in chaos and can roll with those firefighters who feel yoga doesn't belong in the firehouse. I attribute this to years of yoga practice, and it's something I want firefighters to see—that no matter what's going on, you can maintain your focus and inner calm.

Conclusion: Steadiness and Ease

In chapters 8–12, I will walk you through the poses and meditations that instructors generally use for the 10 classes that make up the initial FireFlex Yoga program. In the previous chapter, I explained my 5 themes/10 classes structure, and these chapters follow that plan; each chapter covers one theme and the corresponding two classes. To make these chapters even more user-friendly, each one opens by listing the specific objectives of the classes.

There is no perfect one-size-fits-all sequence for any program, but understanding the mindset of the warrior culture, combined with the patterns of injuries and performance expectations of firefighters, has helped me to design sensible, sustainable yoga sequences. I've carefully focused on *steadiness and ease*, two of the pillars of yoga that are most relevant to first responders. This is the yoga sutra (teaching) underpinning all the classes: "Yoga poses should be stable, and the body be at ease."

Remember the firefighters wearing their CrossFit shoes on their yoga mats? Keep reading and you'll see them gradually get steady in their poses and become at ease as they find the dynamic tension of holding and letting go. Consciously managing pain, listening to their bodies, bringing a distracted mind back to focus, and pushing limits when they feel it's right—in other words, they show grace under fire as practiced on the mat.

Part V

The Classes

8

My Hips Are Too Tight!

CLASSES 1 AND 2

Daily Movement: Flexible hips for walking, running, lunging, and squatting

Functional Fitness Objective: Active straight-leg raise

Interoceptive Awareness: Feeling and identifying a neutral pelvis

Yoga Poses: Pelvic tilts, reclined big toe, low lunge (see chapter 14 for illustrations)

Mindfulness/Meditation: Breathing to activate the relaxation response

---

Too Much Sitting Leads to Pain

In the previous chapter, I described how on day one I often find firefighters standing rather than sitting on their mats. I assumed this was because most firefighters have relatively little experience inside yoga studios and therefore don't understand yoga etiquette. While this is partially true, the more important reason, which I soon discovered, is that sitting on the floor is tough for many of them.

As adults we've grown out of the habit of sitting on floors, an action we found so natural in our youth. Instead, we spend a lot of time sitting at desks or in recliners, couches, kitchen chairs, and car seats. The result? Very tight hips. Specifically, tight adductors and hip flexor muscles, and weak extensors (fig. 8–1).

This is why when firefighters descend to the mats for the first time, it's not that graceful and is generally accompanied by laughter and loud thudding sounds—mostly the sound of them rolling backward as they struggle to find a position that resembles something close to sitting upright. While you will occasionally find firefighters sitting properly, in my experience this is the exception rather than the rule, and the few sitting properly tend to be younger. It may very well be that without the interventions suggested here, these younger firefighters could find themselves in the same situation down the road—all the more reason to start early with yoga!

Tight adductors, hip flexors, and extensors, in addition to weak gluteus muscles, are also prime causes of back pain, one of the most common complaints I hear. At some point in these early classes, I explain that working out at the gym and lifting weights can make tight hips and back pain even worse and can even lead to injury if there's an imbalance

The Pelvic Girdle

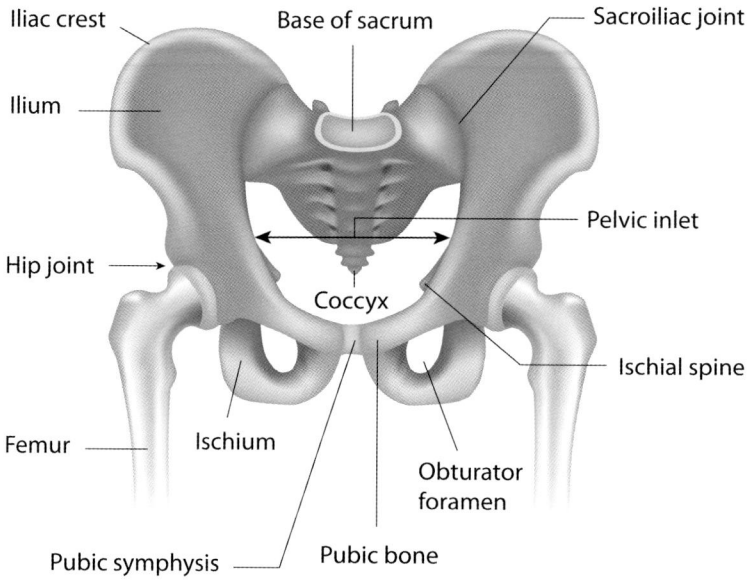

Figure 8–1.
The pelvic girdle and hip
(Image courtesy of Alila Medical Media/Shutterstock.com)

in one's hips. This can be difficult for some firefighters to hear, so I'm very clear that I don't mean you shouldn't work out. I know strength is critical for the work firefighters do. I love the gym and work out myself, so I get it. I'm talking about developing a more balanced workout that looks at total functional movement.

This is the practical reason I start with the hips. There's nothing mystical about practicing a series of poses to open up the hips. You don't have to believe in yoga to feel your hips release. Some of my favorite hip-opening routines can be done lying down, so starting with the hips is super accessible for most firefighters and usually gives some immediate relief of back pain, giving them an incentive to come back for class 2.

Pelvic Stability: The Foundation for Moving Safely

The goal of the poses in classes 1 and 2 is to increase range of motion in the hips. Yet accomplishing this requires understanding the relationship between hips, pelvis, and spine, particularly getting familiar with a balanced pelvis, referred to as *neutral pelvis*. Accordingly, the first pose is usually pelvic tilts.

If your pelvis is balanced in a neutral position, then it's much more stable. With a stable pelvis as a foundation, your hips, spine, neck, and shoulders can more easily go into alignment, and you'll be able to move safely and with better access to your core. This translates to more strength and power when you need it.

The photograph of me with a bowl on my stomach shows what a neutral position looks like (fig. 8–2). The pubic bone and the hip points are in the same plane (vertical when standing, horizontal when lying down) and the right and left hip points are in the same plane. If I tilt my pelvis forward or back too much or rotate one side higher than the other, then the bowl will tilt and the water will spill, indicating that the pelvis is not in a neutral, stable position.

Awareness of pelvic stability is critical for firefighters, especially when the spine is being loaded through heaving lifting. Creating a stable foundation through pelvic stability distributes force throughout the spine in the most optimal and efficient way.

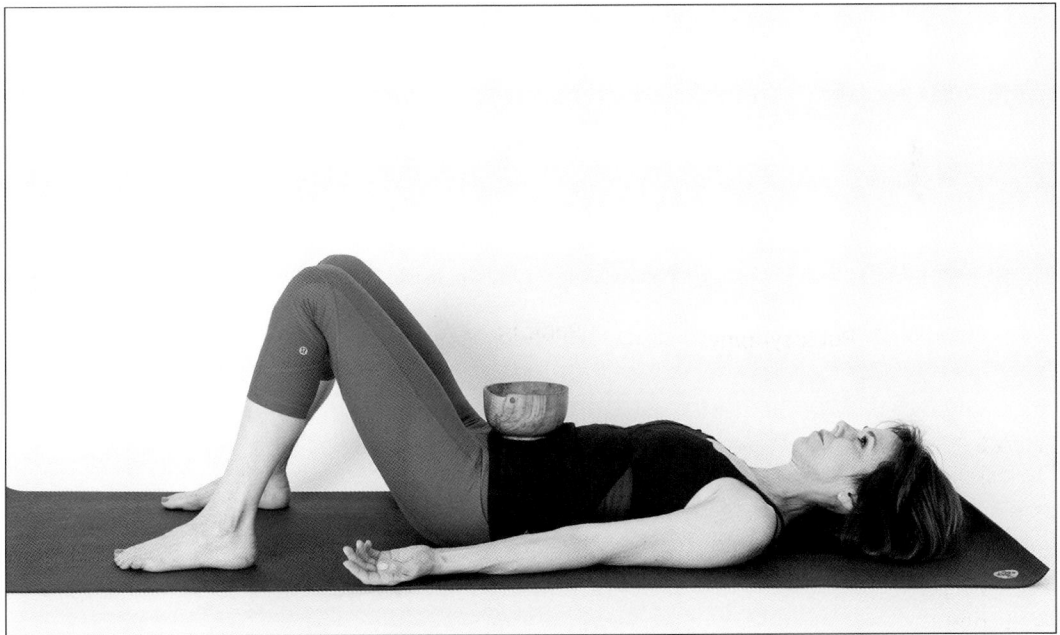

Figure 8–2.
Neutral pelvis

Poses: Pelvic Tilts, Reclined Big Toe, and Low Lunge

Pelvic tilts

Practicing pelvic tilts is a great way to develop an awareness of your neutral position and how to move with that awareness. Here's how you do it: lie on your back with knees bent and feet hip-width apart. Bring your attention to your lower back and the back of your pelvis (the sacrum). Begin to shift your weight toward the tailbone, pressing your tailbone gently into the mat. This action will cause your lower back to lift or feel lighter against the mat. Next curl your tailbone away from the mat, keeping your hips and lower back down, and feel your sacrum and lower back pressing into the mat. Now tilt your pelvis back and forth, pressing your tailbone into the mat and then curling the tailbone away from the mat. Finish this exercise by finding a position for your pelvis that's in between the forward and backward tilt. This will be your neutral (or balanced) pelvis position, a position that will be reinforced in many of the poses found in later chapters.

I don't spend too much time on pelvic tilts in the first few classes because it's a little abstract. After years of practicing, I can feel my pelvis tilting forward or backward when necessary and then moving back to a balanced position. For many firefighters, a neutral pelvis is a new position and can be challenging, especially if their hamstrings or hip flexors are overly tight, making this difficult to even approach. Because I want to keep firefighters from thinking that yoga isn't for them, I keep it simple and just plant seeds to sow in future sessions. Poses like cat, cow, mountain, warrior 2, and half forward fold (see chapter 14) will help firefighters grow into a full awareness of their pelvic position.

Exactly how effective these poses can be was reinforced when my firefighter sister told me about a back injury that happened while she was practicing martial arts. Her back would spasm, making every movement difficult. A great researcher, my sister discovered that to heal her back, she needed to stretch and strengthen all the muscles connected to her pelvis. She came up with a 10–15-minute program she could do at the end of every exercise session, including the yoga poses and stretches in this chapter. As long as she did her exercises, there was no more back pain.

Reclined big toe

This pose is great for stretching the hamstrings, balancing the lower back, and stabilizing the pelvis. With firefighters still lying on their backs, I use a variety of poses to stretch the inner and outer legs. However, to get into this pose, you first have to get hold of your leg.

When I first started working with firefighters, I used my usual yoga studio instructions: "Take your two peace fingers and grab a hold of your right big toe." But when I looked around the room I'd see heads and upper backs suspended off the floor in awkward positions, with some firefighters struggling to grab a hold onto their thighs (forget the big toe), faces pinched in a raisin shape because of the pain.

It took me a few classes to get that they were going to persevere no matter what because that's what I asked them to do, and that's what everyone else was doing. They were simply responding as good firefighters do. Good firefighters make it happen in the face of any obstacle; pain and suffering are part of their duty-before-self mindset. Suggesting to the group that pushing through pain was not necessary on the yoga mat did nothing to change how they responded to the challenges of the poses.

I started bringing enough belts, blocks, and other supports so that every firefighter could use some modification to make the stretches work without pain. If everybody did it, it was okay. Another important point was realizing that any desire on my part to show off would lead the firefighters to redouble their efforts to emulate me, regardless of my edge having 20-plus years of experience.

The important point is that the modifications actually make the pose work. With a strap placed around the ball of one foot, you can move your leg toward straight to stretch tight hamstrings and calf muscles and keep your lower back open. The strap allows your upper back and head to remain on the floor. In addition, keeping the opposite leg bent will allow you to maintain a neutral pelvis (fig. 8-3).

In phase 2 of this hip-opening stretch, you hold the strap in one hand and extend your leg away from your body. This movement produces a stretch to the inner aspect of

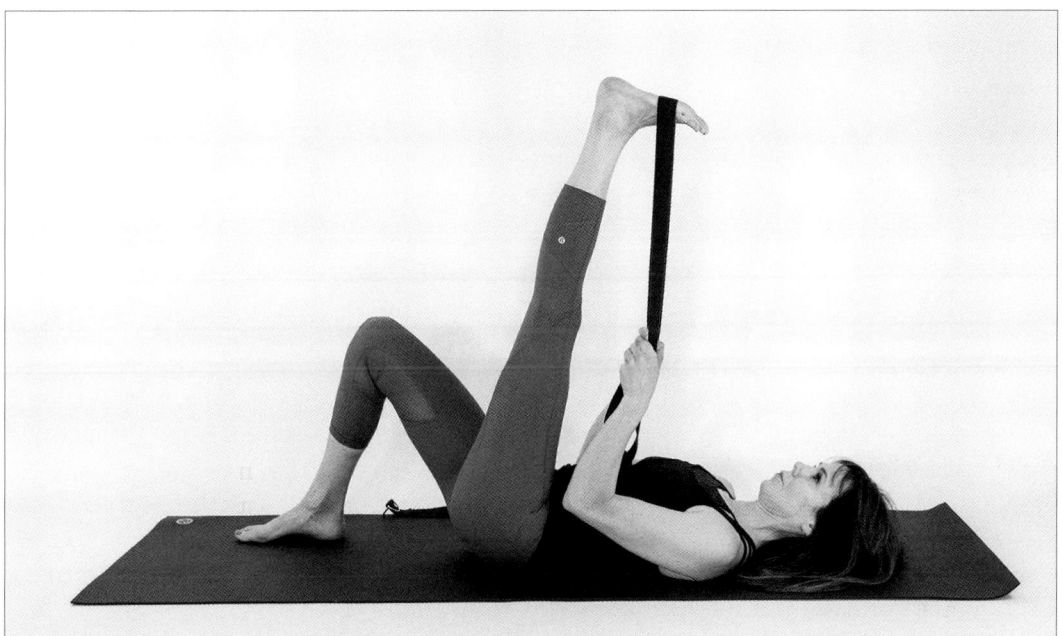

Figure 8–3.
Reclined big toe with strap

the leg and groin on the side of the extended leg. Importantly, to prevent rolling toward the extended leg, you must anchor the opposite side of the pelvis down.

In phase 3, you hold the strap in the opposite hand and draw your leg across your body, stretching the outer hip, iliotibial (IT) band, and gluteus. The IT band of connective tissue runs along the outer thigh, from the top of the pelvis to the shin. By distributing your weight evenly across the back of the pelvis, rather than rolling in the same direction the leg is moving, you'll be able to feel the neutral pelvis position. If you feel any pain or pinching, simply bend the knee of the opposite leg and allow the knee to roll in toward the center of the mat.

Low lunge

Now for the notorious hip flexors! Start in tabletop pose (see chapter 9, page 81). Tent the fingertips (or put blocks under your hands) and move your right foot forward until it is between your hands. Your right knee should be directly above your ankle. Keep the back knee and top of the foot on the mat. Inhale, lift your chest, and bring your hands onto your hips. Tight hip flexors will pull the pelvis forward, so to prevent this, lift the front of your pelvis away from your right thigh and slightly curl your tailbone under. This will help you find a balanced, neutral pelvis. Check that your pelvis is level: front and back, as well as right and left. Switch sides and repeat.

Many firefighters have difficulty stepping the foot forward. Putting blocks under your hands creates more space between your torso and the floor, allowing you to step forward more easily. Also, tight hips can prevent your body weight from being balanced between the front and back legs, causing all the weight to fall on the kneecap. Pressing the kneecap into the floor with this much weight is painful. So another common modification is to put additional padding under that back knee.

No Pain, No Gain

For a yoga teacher, navigating the "no pain, no gain" ethos in a firehouse can be tricky. For that reason, I tell the following story to instructors who are new to fire culture.

During one of my first firehouse yoga classes, I kept paying close attention to a veteran firefighter who was practicing despite many injuries, one of which was a torn anterior cruciate ligament (ACL). However, because he had been cleared to work, it wasn't my job to prevent him from taking yoga classes.

Acutely aware of how fragile his knee was, I kept checking in on him, saying things like "Don't lock your knee," or "Don't bear all your weight on the leg with the injured knee." At one point, I offered him a blanket to provide some cushion for his knee while he was doing a low lunge. This was one suggestion too many, and he finally responded that I was treating him like a baby.

Such attention inside a traditional yoga studio would be accepted and appreciated. I probably wouldn't be questioned if I offered props and tools to make a student's experience more accessible and enjoyable. In the firehouse, though, this extra attention made the injured firefighter feel singled out, not in a good way.

I've had more than one firefighter take only a single class and not return because too many modifications, adjustments, or offering of props was a blow to the ego. Yoga is supposed to be easy, isn't it? When it's not easy—or worse, when firefighters feel awkward because the teacher is providing too much coaching and attention—some of them will not return in order to save face with the rest of the crew. This is one of the many subtleties of teaching yoga to first responders.

Fortunately, there's a happy ending to the story of the firefighter with the torn ACL. He did hang in there for the entire 10 sessions. His awareness of his limited mobility improved, as well as his awareness of how the poses increased or decreased his pain improved. During the course, he learned to safely and incrementally push himself. Eventually, I didn't have to keep an eye on him, because he stopped pushing his body into shapes that caused his entire face to grimace; he proactively applied his own modifications and stayed with the breathing and mindfulness practices throughout every class.

He told me that his reason for joining the classes was to stretch a little and hopefully experience less pain in his knee; he was not prepared for what occurred over the 10 sessions. He said that before doing yoga he was drinking quite heavily, at home and between shifts. When he was drinking he was a bear to be around and gruff with his family. Through yoga classes helping him gain insight into his behavior, he realized he was using alcohol to cope with his situation, which was generating more problems for him. Now, he was using the yoga stretches and breathing practices at home, drinking less, and enjoying his family more.

Diaphragmatic Breathing

The goal of the relaxation and breathing exercises for classes 1 and 2 is to experience the relationship between *diaphragmatic breathing* and activation of the parasympathetic nervous system. (Chapter 4 explained that this system is the main pathway for calming the sympathetic nervous system to reduce stress and bring the body back to homeostasis. The breath is one of the fastest, most effective ways to do this.) Also, diaphragmatic breathing massages the spine and can reduce lower back pain.

Yoga breathing practices can be quite complex and may feel unnatural for many firefighters. For instance, learning how to relax the abdomen as you inhale, rather than sucking in the belly, can make you feel awkward or vulnerable. In the spirit of increasing mind and body awareness in a way that's respectful to firefighters newer to practice, I don't belabor the role of diaphragmatic breathing to activate the vagus nerve. Instead, I encourage firefighters to simply notice how their bodies move as they breathe.

Here's an example you can try: start by lying on your back. Place one hand on your sternum and the other on your abdomen. Without altering your breath, notice which hand moves more as you breathe. Most likely, at least initially, the hand on your sternum will move more.

Next, for the second phase of this practice, keep your hands over your abdomen. On inhalation, press your abdomen into your hands and feel the hand lift. On exhalation, do the opposite and press your hand into your abdomen, feeling it move toward your spine. Now, simply focus on the sensations in your abdomen, or the pressure of your hands against it.

During class we'll do this practice for one to two minutes. While explaining how to engage the diaphragm with respiration, I talk briefly about how important this kind of breathing is for firefighters. By contrast, chest breathing is inefficient because the breath is shallow. It's how we breathe when we're stressed. Diaphragmatic (or abdominal) breathing is more efficient because when the diaphragm contracts, it pulls and opens the lower lungs, producing greater gas exchange—more air, in other words. Ever watch a baby or a loved one sleeping? Their abdomens move as they breathe, because abdominal breathing is the way we breathe when sleeping or relaxed.

Breathing techniques with self-contained breathing apparatus

Efficient breath regulation is crucial when you need to use a self-contained breathing apparatus (SCBA) to get air. Air bottles last longer when you slow down and regulate your breath. During this part of the class, I often share a story from my friend Fire Chief David Dolson.

As mentioned previously, Dolson is a certified yoga instructor. In the line of duty, he uses his breath to keep himself as calm and focused as possible when dispatched to an emergency call. Consequently, when the tones go off and a ton of information starts coming in, Dolson is able to focus on all that information, to make good decisions about the crew's response.

When Chief Dolson gets to an emergency scene and has to use the SCBA, he uses the following process: when he notices he's breathing faster than he would like, or his breathing is becoming shallow or rapid, he says to himself, "Okay, breathe." Then he starts the breath work he learned in yoga to bring himself back into balance. Here's how he explained it to me: "As I'm exerting myself and moving around the fire/emergency scene with all this equipment on and helping my firefighters advance the hose line and fight the fire, I'm able to keep a nice consistent breath. I might be breathing faster than normal, but it's balanced rather than agitated. This is now a habitual muscle memory process that has become very valuable to my profession." What Dolson is talking about is directly in line with good practices for better situational awareness.

A Yoga Superstar Learns How to Sit on the Ground

My own yoga teacher, Mark Stephens, had at one point found sitting on the floor with legs crossed so uncomfortable for him that he started by sitting on top of several phone books. Day after day, week by week, he would rip out pages of one of the books, several at a time. Slowly, the muscles surrounding his hips and pelvis began to relax and release until eventually he was sitting on the floor. This process probably took six months or longer.

As a suggestion for the digital age, in which phone books are no longer readily available, try the following exercise to help you sit on the floor comfortably: at the firehouse or at home, instead of sitting on the couches or recliners, sit on the floor. You can use an old beach towel or mat. And if station floors are not conducive, then you can do the following practices when you are at home. Use furniture to support your back. Press down through the base of your pelvis and gently lift and extend (lengthen) your spine. Over time, feel the weight of your body move from the tailbone toward the front of your sit bones (ischial tuberosity). Gradually feel the back of your pelvis tilt toward your lumbar spine.

Conclusion

After only one or two classes, most firefighters experience some relief from tight hips and other sore, constricted muscles. As they feel more movement in their joints and a release of tension in their bodies, their enthusiasm for yoga practice skyrockets.

I remember teaching an early morning class before the Training Chiefs Conference in Central California. The first two classes were advertised to release tight hips and shoulders. A fire chief came up to me at the beginning of the second class and told me how much better his back felt after just one session. He demonstrated how easily he could rotate his torso in one direction and then the other while standing. The big smile on his face about his new-found freedom of movement is one of the great joys I get from teaching these classes.

At the end of the 10 classes, we look for quantifiable improvements in FMS scores and stress assessments (see chapter 6). For the long term, we want firefighters to stay enthusiastic and committed to a regular practice both on and off duty. A long-term commitment will help them experience the transformative aspects of yoga and improve their job performance through better functional and mental fitness. Primarily, after classes 1 and 2, we're just thrilled to have everyone experiencing some pain relief and coming back for classes 3 and 4!

9

Shouldering the Burden

CLASSES 3–4

Daily Movement: Mobile shoulders for reaching, lifting, pulling, and dragging

Functional Fitness Objective: Shoulder mobility test, shoulder impingement clearing test

Interoceptive Awareness: Feeling and identifying external rotation and rhomboid activation, healthy placement of the shoulders before loading the joint

Yoga Poses: Supine chest stretch, tabletop, mountain, cow face (see chapter 14 for illustrations)

Mindfulness/Meditation: Box breathing

Get to Know Your Infraspinatus and Teres Muscles

After years of working in the fire service, I've learned that many shoulder injuries originate because firefighters are unaware of the position of the shoulder joint before loading it. Consider the examples of removing heavy equipment from your vehicle, lifting a heavy person onto a stretcher, or pulling down a ceiling. In each of these cases, if your shoulder joint is in an internally rotated position (fig. 9–1), rather than externally rotated (fig. 9–2), you've just set yourself up for possible injury—or for aggravating an already sore shoulder.

As a first responder, you sometimes have no choice but to operate in an uncomfortable or awkward position. Usually, however, it's simply a matter of awareness. For example, before you pick up a patient, take a moment to adjust your shoulders.

This lack of awareness is not limited to firefighters. A good percentage of the general population walks around with internally rotated shoulder joints. Modern life isn't helping. Too much driving, texting, and keyboarding, as well as standing and sitting in a slumped position, cause us to round our upper backs and shoulders.

Adding to the challenge for firefighters are already-tight pectoralis (pecs) and latissimus dorsi (lats) muscles that come from lifting weights. Often weightlifters talk about pumping up their pecs and lats, but when's the last time you heard someone say, "I'm gonna pump up my infraspinatus and teres minor." Probably never, right? They don't even have catchy names.

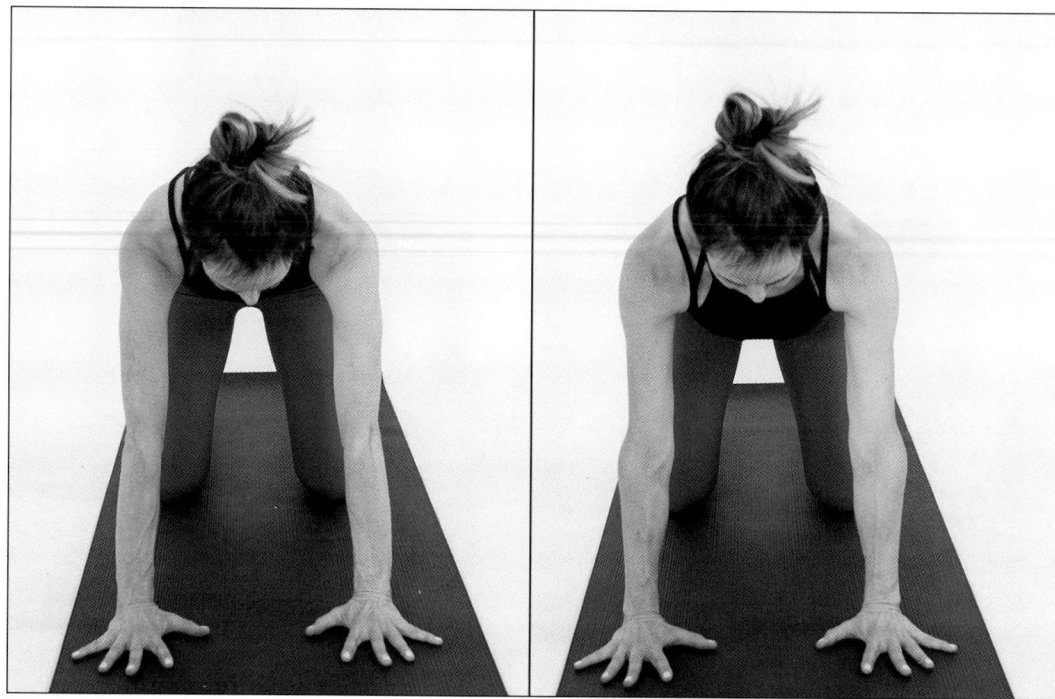

Figure 9–1.
Internally rotated shoulder position

Figure 9–2.
Externally rotated shoulder position

Here's the problem: pecs and lats are the internal shoulder rotators, and infraspinatus and teres minor muscles are the external shoulder rotators. Training programs that focus primarily on pecs and lats (as are common) can contribute to an imbalance between the internal and external rotator muscle groups, which in combination with habitual slumping and shoulder rounding can lead to shortened internal rotators and weak external rotators. As a result, the shoulder joint no longer has the strength and stability it needs to perform efficiently when you load it.

Upper-crossed syndrome is an example of what can happen when the head and shoulders are extended forward. When the head pulls forward, the shoulders round, causing impingement in the shoulders and reduced mobility in the thoracic spine (the chest area). This syndrome can cause headaches, upper back pain, sprains and strains, rotator cuff tears, and even bone spurs in the neck and shoulder. For firefighters, this syndrome can affect job performance because of pain and movement impairment.

Shoulder pain is tricky, and a serious injury needs medical attention and perhaps physical therapy. Make sure your therapist works with you on the exercises that are part of your typical routine. Yoga, which has a great track record for alleviating shoulder pain from overuse, muscle imbalances, and bad posture, complements other therapies. Further, certain yoga routines that require repetitive movements, such as the four-limbed staff pose (Chaturanga Dandasana), can take a toll on the healthiest of shoulder joints over time. The primary movement goal of classes 3 and 4 is to stretch the internal rotators, strengthen external rotators, and help firefighters become aware of when their shoulders are in the proper position to avoid injury, which is a slightly externally rotated position.

Balancing shoulder mobility and stability

As explained in chapter 6, good functional movement requires a yin-yang balance of mobility and stability. Getting this right is particularly difficult with the shoulder because it's the most flexible joint in the body, making it intrinsically less stable and therefore more prone to injury. Figure 9–3 shows that the shoulder is a ball-and-socket joint. The ball at the top end of the arm bone (humerus) fits into the small socket (glenoid) of the shoulder blade (scapula) to form the shoulder joint, the rotator cuff encircles the top of the humerus, and the collarbone (clavicle) connects the shoulder blades to the upper part of the breastbone (sternum). With so many moving parts and the flexibility to rotate 180°, shoulders are both a wonder and an injury magnet.

A few hundred firefighters have taken the FMS (see chapter 6) before taking their first FireFlex Yoga class. I use the results from the shoulder mobility exercises to design classes 3 and 4. Figure 9–4 shows me giving the reciprocal reaching exercise.

Many of the firefighters I work with report pain in the shoulder that is adducting and internally rotating (moving the arm to the middle of the body). They also report experiencing *asymmetry*, meaning one shoulder is moving better than the other. As part of the shoulder mobility screen, firefighters perform the impingement clearing test, which is particularly good for spotting minor rotator cuff injuries. That pain is frequently reported while performing this test indicates that a lot of problems with rotator cuffs are going undetected and untreated.

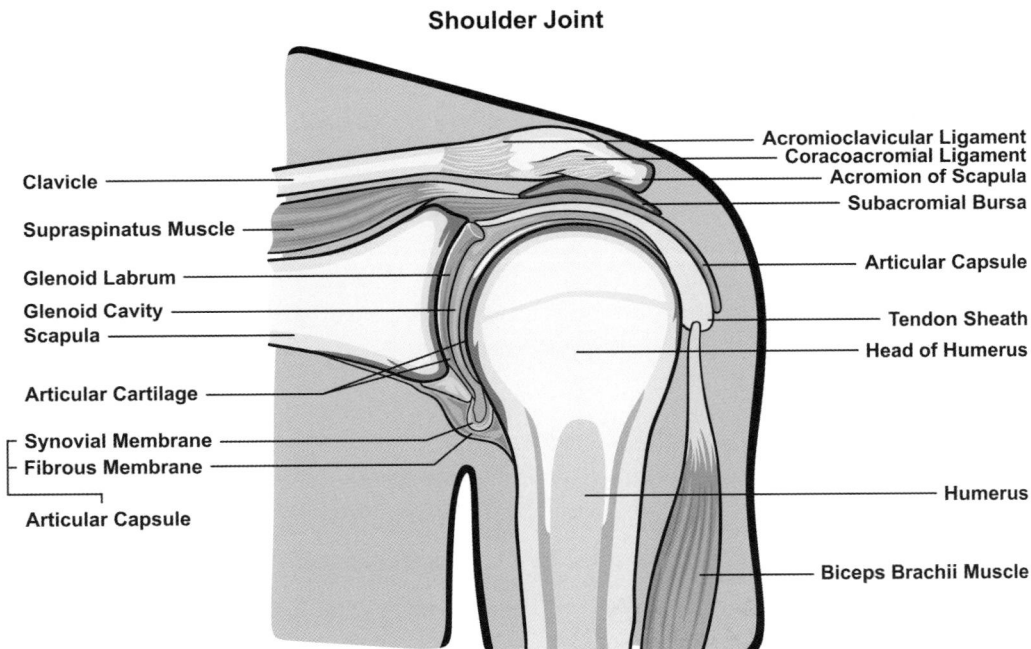

Figure 9–3.
Shoulder joint
(Image courtesy of Adaix/Shutterstock.com)

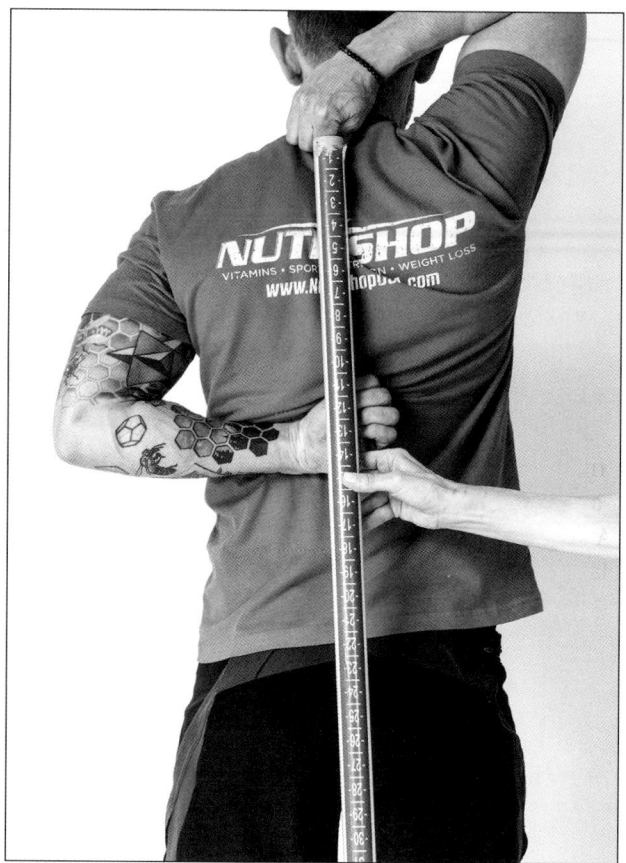

Figure 9–4.
Reciprocal reaching exercise

There is also the fact that we have two shoulders—again, the asymmetry problem. Before we even start the shoulder mobility screen, most firefighters will say something like, "Oh, this shoulder is going to be bad!" They already know there's a difference in pain and movement from shoulder to shoulder that correlates to their dominant hand. In my experience, right-handed firefighters report more problems with their right shoulder and left-handed firefighters with their left shoulder, when the shoulders are internally rotated and adducting. So the additional challenge for classes 3 and 4 is to reduce this lopsidedness many firefighters are living with.

Poses: Supine Chest Stretch, Tabletop, and Mountain

This sequence of poses stretches and opens the muscles of the chest, activates the muscles in between the shoulder blades, and strengthens the muscles of the upper back so they can pull the fronts of the shoulders back. In other words, it is getting in the right position for externally rotated shoulder joints. There are a number of other effective poses for shoulders, and I sometimes vary this sequence; however, I've found that these three are particularly good for the kinds of overhead reaching and pulling movements firefighters do all the time. Even being rigorous enough for regular yoga practitioners, they're also accessible for beginners.

I start both classes 3 and 4 with the firefighters on their backs, doing diaphragmatic breathing using the techniques learned in classes 1 and 2. This helps everyone start the process of slowing down from their busy and often chaotic schedules and turning their attention to what's happening in their bodies. Initially, there will be dissonance between what everyone is feeling right before diaphragmatic breathing and the sensations that come after. It's a strange feeling because within moments of lying on their backs and focusing on their breath, firefighters are suddenly aware of the tremendous tension and stress they've been holding in their necks and shoulders that wasn't detectable just moments before. One of yoga's greatest gifts for firefighters is interoception!

While focusing on the breath, we take a couple of minutes to regain awareness of the position of the hips and neutral pelvis, then start moving that awareness to the position of the shoulder joints and upper back. There's a definite cause-and-effect relationship between tight hips and tight shoulders, so just bringing this awareness readies the body for the first pose. Although awareness of the neutral pelvis takes time and practice to develop, after one class, firefighters are already learning how to bend their knees to decompress the lower back or make similar adjustments without my prompting.

Supine chest stretch

This stretch opens the shoulder in an uploaded position. Start by lying on your left side with left arm extended on the floor (at the height of the shoulder), palm facing toward the ceiling, and right palm stacking on top of the left. On inhalation, slowly lift your right arm and stretch it in an arc up toward the ceiling. Let your head move along with your arm. Continue moving your right arm and head behind you and toward the floor, as far as you can comfortably go. For firefighters who have enough flexibility in the internal rotators and chest, their right arm and hand will come far enough down so the knuckles touch the floor. Then slowly lift the arm back up toward the ceiling and down to starting position. Repeat a few times, then switch sides.

If you try this pose, you might run into the same problem as many of the firefighters in class. Tight chest muscles and internal rotators on the moving arm prevent almost everyone from getting their arms far enough down to touch the floor. Their arms end up suspended in the air. Anticipating this kind of challenge, I have blocks or blankets ready so firefighters can modify the position and relax the arm. After they try the stretch a few more times, they start to feel the muscles loosening and the raised arm slowly releasing downward, a bit farther with each repetition. The interoceptive learning here is, "This is as far as I can go right now." The goal is not touching the ground; instead it's awareness of the body and the limitations of the movement—learning to do the movement without forcing it.

Tabletop pose

After opening up the upper chest, we move to the tabletop position, which I particularly like for firefighters because it allows them to practice external rotation of the shoulders safely. Start on your hands and knees, wrists under shoulders and knees under hips. Next, create a slight bend in your elbows, and turn the inner crease of the elbows forward. This draws the triceps back and the biceps forward. Feel the collarbones broaden and the shoulder blades spread across and down the back. This action frees the neck. Practicing this simple but powerful movement starts to strengthen the external rotators, which stabilizes the scapula to maintain proper shoulder positioning.

Most firefighters get the hang of this movement quickly. Still, I like to wait for the aha moment when they realize that they can keep their shoulders externally rotated while their lower arms have the freedom to rotate for actions like pulling equipment from the truck. Most importantly, they can then perform these actions in the line of duty without compromising their shoulders (fig. 9–5).

In class 3, I begin mentioning that top athletes, especially those who play overhead sports, practice this opposite rotation to prevent injuries. Another key point I build on throughout the program is how the whole body works together. An article in the journal *Sports Medicine* elaborates on this idea: "Core stability is defined as the ability to control the position and motion of the trunk over the pelvis to allow optimum production, transfer and control of force and motion to the terminal segment in integrated athletic activities."[1] Put simply, if athletes or first responders want to run, throw, reach, and lift safely and with optimum efficiency, then they need to develop the core strength to stabilize the pelvis and trunk. This is one of the reasons I start with the hips and pelvis in classes 1 and 2.

Mountain pose

Mountain pose continues to strengthen the awareness of keeping the shoulders externally rotated because standing is a pose we do all the time. Start standing tall, feet hip distance apart or wide enough to feel stable. Begin stretching your fingertips toward your toes. Begin to rotate both thumbs and palms outward. As you continue to rotate your palms

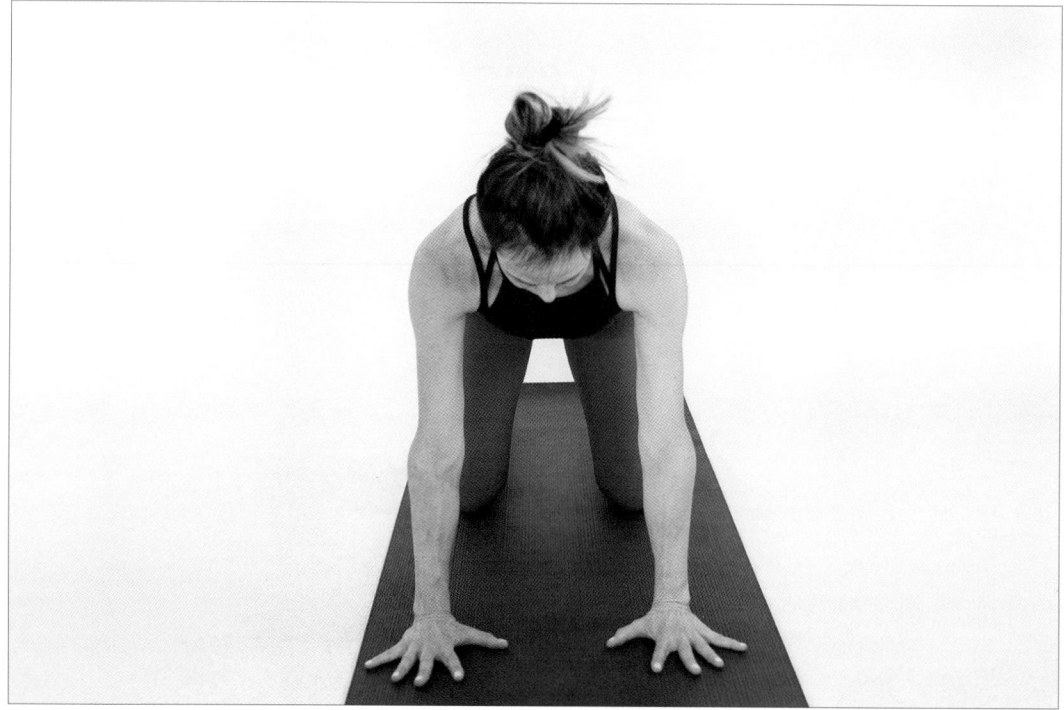

Figure 9–5.
Externally rotated shoulder with neutral lower arm

outward, feel your forearms rotate away from the thighs while the biceps, in the upper arms, move the forearms into external rotation. You should feel your shoulder blades retracting or moving toward each other as you activate the rhomboids (the muscles that pull your shoulder blades together). Next, keeping a nice opposite rotation with biceps moving forward and triceps moving back, take your arms overhead with the palms facing each other, moving into extended mountain pose. Make sure to breathe, relaxing the tops of the shoulders and shoulder blades so they extend or move away and slide over the back of the rib cage.

Reciprocal reaching stretch with strap (optional)

If most of the firefighters in a particular group scored low in the reciprocal reaching exercise section of the FMS, I'll add this pose. Here's the challenge: with one arm reaching over your shoulder, palm touching the upper back and fingers facing down, and the other arm reaching around the waist, palm touching the lower back and fingers facing up, try to interlace your fingers. During class there's usually a lot of muttering and grimacing, and most firefighters have a one- to two-foot space between hands. Once again, rotators are the root of the problem: weak external rotators that inhibit the upper arm movement, and tight internal rotators that inhibit the lower arm movement. By now firefighters are getting more comfortable with modifications, so they use straps to help them relax into the position and bring the hands closer together (fig. 9–6).

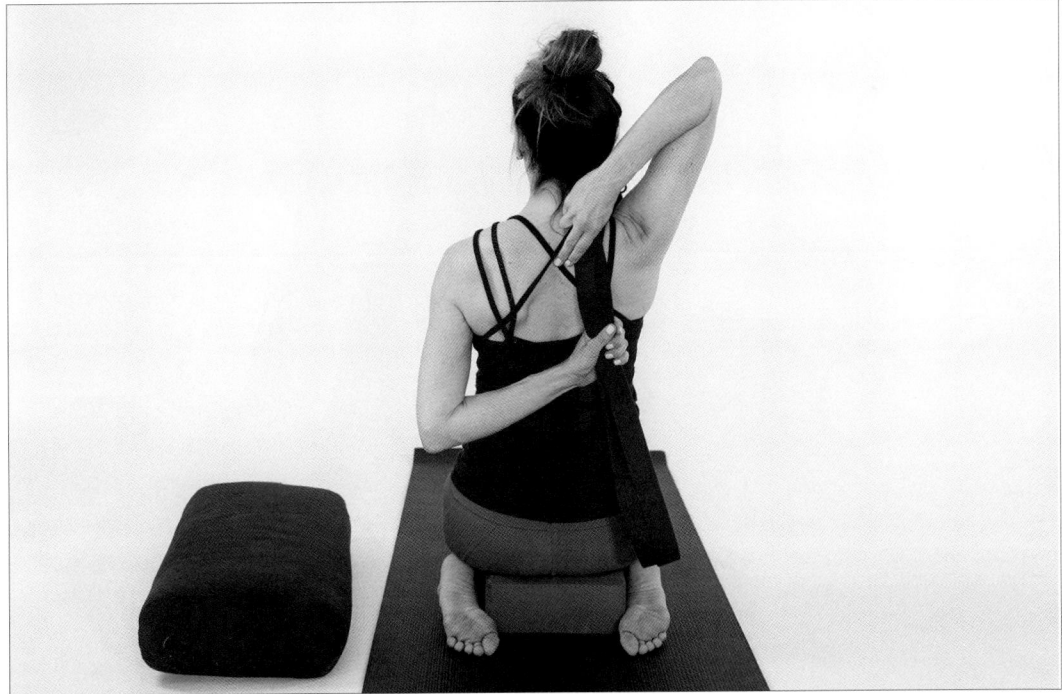

Figure 9–6.
Reciprocal reach modification

Box Breathing

After doing poses for 40–50 minutes and becoming aware of the sensations produced by the different positions, everyone's mind is more grounded and prepared to focus on breathing exercises. An additional problem with chronically rounded shoulders is constriction of the chest, which makes efficient breathing more difficult. Thus, in classes 3 and 4, we expand on diaphragmatic breathing and mind-body integration by adding a technique called *box breathing*. This is a counting practice that is very popular among tactical professionals like military and first responders—hence its other name, combat breathing. One police officer credits it for saving her life after getting shot, calling it a "mandatory component of survival stress management."[2]

In box breathing, the breath is divided into four stages or phases:

1. Inhalation
2. Breath retention
3. Exhalation
4. Breath retention

All four phases are practiced for the same length of time. I typically use four seconds for each phase: inhale for four seconds, hold for four seconds, exhale for four seconds, and hold for four seconds.

Here are the instructions if you'd like to try: start by lying on your back. To prepare, breathe in deeply for a count of four, then exhale audibly with your mouth open. Now, close your mouth and inhale for 1-2-3-4, hold the breath for 1-2-3-4, exhale for 1-2-3-4, and hold with the lungs empty of air for 1-2-3-4; then begin again. I usually lead four to six cycles and then ask firefighters to continue for several more cycles, silently counting by themselves.

Box breathing is not as easy as it appears because breathing is relatively unconscious and we rarely retain our breath. Nevertheless, it's a great way to reduce stress when you're in fight-or-flight mode and to focus the mind to react calmly to the situation at hand. Thus, practicing on the mat gives firefighters a chance to get comfortable with using the breath consciously. Later, they can use their breath awareness to assist them in a crisis.

Visualization

We do Savasana for the final three to five minutes of class. While encouraging everyone to relax and let the body and mind integrate the learning from the class, I often give a short visualization or suggestion to become aware of their breathing and take in the sensations around them.

You can experiment with this power of awareness by taking a moment to listen to the sounds in your environment. Most likely you can hear sounds that your brain had blocked out. The sounds don't suddenly appear because you start to listen. But once you start to listen, you can hear them. When you pay attention to your breath, an entire world of thoughts, feelings and sensations can be detected simply because you choose to pay attention. As renowned trauma specialist Dr. Bessel van der Kolk says, "As long as you keep secrets and suppress information, you are fundamentally at war with yourself . . . The critical issue is allowing yourself to know what you know. That takes an enormous amount of courage."[3]

10

Trunk Stability for Your Aching Back

Daily Movement: Stable trunk for lifting, twisting, carrying, and chopping

Functional Fitness Objective: Trunk stability push-up, rotary stability, extension and flexion clearing tests

Interoceptive Awareness: Stabilizing the spine against movement

Yoga Poses: Stomach turning, plank, downward-facing dog (see chapter 14 for illustrations)

Mindfulness/Meditation: Ujjayi warrior breathing

Turning up the Heat: Activating the Core

What is it about developing core strength that takes so much will and effort? Most likely it's because most of us are not very connected to our core and neglect to exercise those muscles (except for the rectus abdominis to achieve those six-pack abs!). In every yoga studio I've ever been in, when the teacher says, usually with great enthusiasm, "Now we're going to focus on the core," there's a universal groan. But there's no getting away from it. If you visualize the core as the "central link in a chain connecting your upper and lower body," you'll get an idea of how important this area is to how your whole body moves.[1]

Groans aside, in classes 5 and 6, I turn up the heat with poses that activate and strengthen the core. A stable core protects your spine and maintains trunk stability while you move. Therefore, strong core muscles are especially important for firefighters and other tactical athletes who regularly load their bodies with 60+ pounds of gear. Weak core muscles, by contrast, can lead to less endurance, more fatigue, and susceptibility to muscle injuries and back pain—major issues for firefighters.[2]

The trunk stability push-up

This is one of the toughest diagnostic exercises in the FMS. Firefighters think it's going to be easy—like a traditional push-up. But although the two look similar, with the trunk stability push-up we're gauging the ability of the spine to stabilize (not move) through the entire range of motion. In other words, how well does the trunk—pelvis, spine, and shoulders—move together as one unit?

In this pose, the thumbs need to line up with the forehead for men or with the chin for women. You can't muscle through this test with bicep and shoulder strength. This is why this falls in the sequence as it does—after classes 1 and 2 to increase mobility in the hips and classes 3 and 4 to increase mobility in the shoulders. Only with proper mobility or range of motion in the hips can you achieve a stable pelvis and lower back—and only with proper mobility in the shoulders can you build stability in the upper back.

What happens, though, if you're not so good at doing the trunk stability push-up? It may be surprising, but this is the case for the majority of firefighters taking the FMS. They either underperform because of weak trunk stability or can't do the pose at all because of shoulder pain. This is where the will comes in. Do you power through it, collapse and give up, or end up somewhere in between?

Not doing well with poses requiring core strength is particularly frustrating for firefighters who thought yoga would be easy. I've heard many firefighters who didn't succeed at a pose discount either yoga or their teacher. This attitude, by the way, is a good example of a fixed mindset (see chapter 3). Essentially, strengthening the core is often where the rubber meets the road—or the mat.

Activating the Will the Conscious Warrior Way

Yoga can illuminate our reflexive behavior patterns in the face of challenges and teach us a lot about our will and the emotions that get activated when our sense of power and control is threatened. It just so happens that in yoga, the core corresponds to our third *chakra*, or energy center. This energy center, located around the solar plexus, is connected with our personal power and will; it influences our self-confidence, agency, and ability to achieve goals. Remember that yoga has a 5,000-year history as an enlightened warrior practice, so don't get taken in by assumptions that it's for people who are built like Olive Oyl instead of Popeye.

Particularly for first responders, practicing these more challenging poses is a safe way to take risks and recognize limitations with few consequences. It's a way to develop a more open mindset and the habit of consciously modulating the will: when to fall out of a pose, how to modify it, and when to get back in it.

Ultimately, a certain amount of stress or friction is what allows us to expand our skills and grow as a person and as a leader. When we stress muscle tissue, the body sends more blood and oxygen to those tissues so they become stronger and can handle even more pressure, stress, or friction over time. This same analogy can be applied to your core muscles as well as your nervous system. When you hold poses longer than you thought possible, when you can invoke a calm, steady breath while your body is quaking and shaking, you grow your capacity to handle difficult sensations and emotions. You can now handle these sensations and emotions without becoming overwhelmed. This is a more conscious, self-aware employment of the will; it stands in contrast to automatically powering through pain, denying vulnerability at any cost. One of the benefits of regular yoga practice is becoming more centered, grounded, confident, and bold during chaos and challenge.

Speaking from Experience

I discovered yoga after my motorcycle and I had an unfortunate encounter with a very large automobile. I was 26 years old at the time of the accident and in a lot of pain as I worked hard to recover (years later I'm still dealing with neck and jaw problems). I was facing a possible hip replacement, and doctors told me I had to stop running, my primary form of stress release, as well as give up skiing.

None of those options sounded good to me. Physical therapy was very helpful and got me part of the way to recovery. However, when I found yoga, I started building a new relationship with my body. I began listening and paying attention to my body rather than treating it like an inconvenience that needed to be fed and exercised. Developing core strength and trunk stability through yoga helped me develop patience (not one of my primary attributes!) and a willingness to try something new. With time and dedicated practice, I was able to slow down and experience how the five minutes of complete relaxation at the end of every yoga class was more than just nap time. This was the recovery time needed for my nervous system to find homeostasis, or balance, and for my body and mind to integrate the new physical and mental habits I was developing. Years later, I still have the same hip! I do sports and perform strenuous exercises and yoga poses almost daily. Recovery didn't happen overnight, but it did happen.

Over the years, yoga has taught me a lot about recovery. Not just long-term recovery from an accident or illness, but the short, microrecovery moments we all need in order to deal with the stress of everyday life. Tony Schwartz is an international thought leader building more humane, higher-performing organizations, workings with top athletes, executives, and entire organizations such as Coca-Cola and Google. About recovery, Schwartz says, "The real enemy is not stress. . . . Rather, the problem is the absence of disciplined, intermittent recovery. Chronic stress without recovery leads to burnout and breakdown, and ultimately undermines performance."[3] Read the sidebar for two of his tips for being more productive. Notice the parallels with yoga!

Recovery Tips

These two tips are from Tony Schwartz's article "Six Ways to Supercharge Your Productivity."

- *Live like a sprinter, not a marathoner.* When you work continuously, you're actually progressively depleting your energy reservoir as the day wears on. By making intermittent renewal and refueling important, you're regularly replenishing your reservoir, so you're not only able to fully engage at intervals along the way, but also to maintain high energy much further into the day.
- *Monitor your mood.* When demand begins to exceed your capacity, one of the most common signs is an increase in negative emotions. The more we move into "fight-or-flight," the more reactive and impulsive we become, and the less reflective and responsive. The first question to ask yourself is "Why am I feeling this way, and what can I do to make myself feel better?" It may be that you're hungry, tired, overwhelmed, or feeling threatened in some way. Awareness is the first step. You can't change what you don't notice.[4]

Poses: Stomach Turning, Plank, and Downward-Facing Dog

This sequence is particularly good for beginning yoga students because it provides a safe way to build both strength and stability from the core through the entire trunk. The risk is gradually increased: initially, the floor supports much of the body's weight, with the trunk eventually taking over the job.

Stomach turning

This pose is done lying on your back. It is my go-to posture for waking up the core (especially obliques) and bringing awareness to the trunk before going into plank and side plank. This is important because firefighters are vulnerable to shoulder and back injuries, both of which can be exacerbated in typical yoga core-strengthening poses.

Try this pose now. Lying on your back, knees bent and feet planted, feel your entire upper spine pressing into the mat. Note the position of your chin and adjust it to support the natural curve of your neck; also note the position of your pelvis and adjust it to support the natural curve of your lower back. Draw your shoulder blades together gently to release the fronts of your shoulders toward the mat and spread your collarbones. The spine is now properly oriented in the body and supported by the floor, and you should now exhale and lift your feet off the floor and bring your knees directly above your hips. Next, place a block between your knees and press on the block with the knees. Extend your arms out creating a T shape with your torso, and as you continue squeezing the block, gently rock your knees from side to side, keeping your shoulders and upper back on the mat. Become aware of the rotation of your lower back as you lower your knees from one side to the other. Only lower your knees as long as it is comfortable for your lower back. The action of squeezing the block activates the pelvic floor and deep core muscles. An option you can try is to roll your head in the opposite direction from your knees. If you have a neck injury or neck pain, consult with your doctor before you attempt this.

While rotation is contraindicated for anyone with a sacroiliac joint dysfunction, many firefighters feel tremendous relief from this movement. One of the challenges for firefighters is balancing upper body stability with lower body mobility. Upper body stability also allows for safe rotation of the lower spine. The interoceptive learning in the pose is to pay attention to the rotation of the spine and to lower the knees only as far as you can while keeping the opposite shoulder and shoulder blade pressing into the mat.

Plank

With plank, the risk of failure increases, which makes it a chance to face your shadow side (see chapter 1). One of the big challenges is tight quadriceps (thigh muscles) that pull the pelvis into a forward tilt and cause the pelvis to sag, putting excessive pressure on the lower back. For this reason, I have students start in tabletop (see chapter 9). Once you get into tabletop, there are two important points: make sure your shoulders are externally rotated, with shoulder blades stabilized on the back; and check that your pelvis and spine are aligned. Remember, a neutral pelvis supports a stable spine.

Now you're ready to step back into plank. Your spine is resisting the downward pull of gravity. Your shoulders, pelvis, and ankles should be lined up on a diagonal.

What I typically see from new students, however, is sagging pelvises (fig. 10–1). To reduce the sag, work your legs strongly, activating your quadriceps, and press through your heels. Then slightly tuck your tailbone to engage your lower abdomen and lift the front of your body away from the mat.

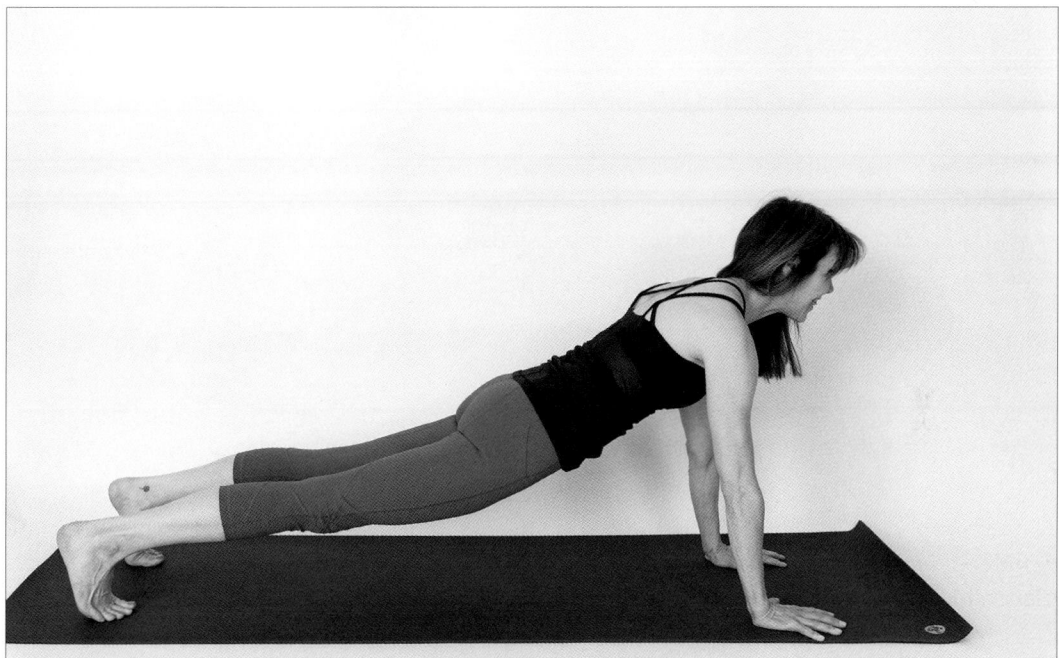

Figure 10–1.
Sagging pelvis during plank

Downward-facing dog

Downward-facing dog is deservedly one of yoga's most popular poses because it energizes and awakens every part of the body as well as gently decompressing the spine. It also presents a number of challenges. It takes a stable core to support flexion in the shoulders and hips, and staying in it for any length of time tests even experienced yoga practitioners. That said, watching firefighters take on the challenge, find their modifications, and gradually own the pose inspires my own practice.

With sufficient trunk stability, downward-facing dog can be done starting in plank. Otherwise the knees can be lowered. Plank is a good preliminary pose to downward-facing dog because the feet and hands are spaced properly.

Starting from plank, root down through your palms and separate your feet hip-width apart. Take a deep breath in and as you exhale slightly bend your knees and lift your pelvis up and back. The tendency will be to walk your hands closer to your feet to find power in your shoulders and upper back. If you find that happening, use your legs as leverage. Press the upper legs strongly back and root down through the balls of your feet. If your heels are lifting away from the mat, consider rolling the mat under your feet to bring your heels closer to the floor.

The challenges for firefighters in downward-facing dog are numerous, so I'll focus on the two most important. The first challenge comes from the upper body. When performed properly and safely, downward-facing dog takes strong, stable shoulder joints capable of external rotation with weight. Firefighters typically have upper body strength, but their focus is usually on biceps and pecs. If they don't have the necessary shoulder strength, they tend to muscle through using their biceps and pecs.

Unfortunately, these are the very muscles they need to release to find external rotation. Recruiting the biceps and pecs causes the shoulders to internally rotate and the shoulder blades to retract and slide toward the neck, compressing the upper spine. This can cause neck and back pain. One modification that can be done initially, while building up your shoulder stability, is to bend your elbows slightly and rotate the eye of each elbow toward the top of your yoga mat (so your elbows are not pointing out to the side).

Now imagine you are squeezing a large beach ball in between your elbows and in front of your face. As you squeeze this imaginary beach ball, start to straighten your arms. The pressure you want to feel will be around the outer edge of your armpits. See Figures 10–2 and 10–3 for examples of good and bad downward-facing dog poses.

The second important challenge comes from the lower body. Because of their lifestyle, firefighters tend to have very tight hips and weak gluteus muscles (glutes). The pelvis should be able to tilt slightly forward while moving up and back, but tight hamstrings prevent this rotation. For firefighters with this problem, their downward-facing dog looks like a plank pose with a hump, rather than an upside-down V, as it should. One modification is to bend the knees and open up the feet the width of the mat.

Importantly, it's not strength that gets you into downward-facing dog. Instead, it's moderate effort over time that develops both strength and flexibility. It's a deeper, more balanced strength.

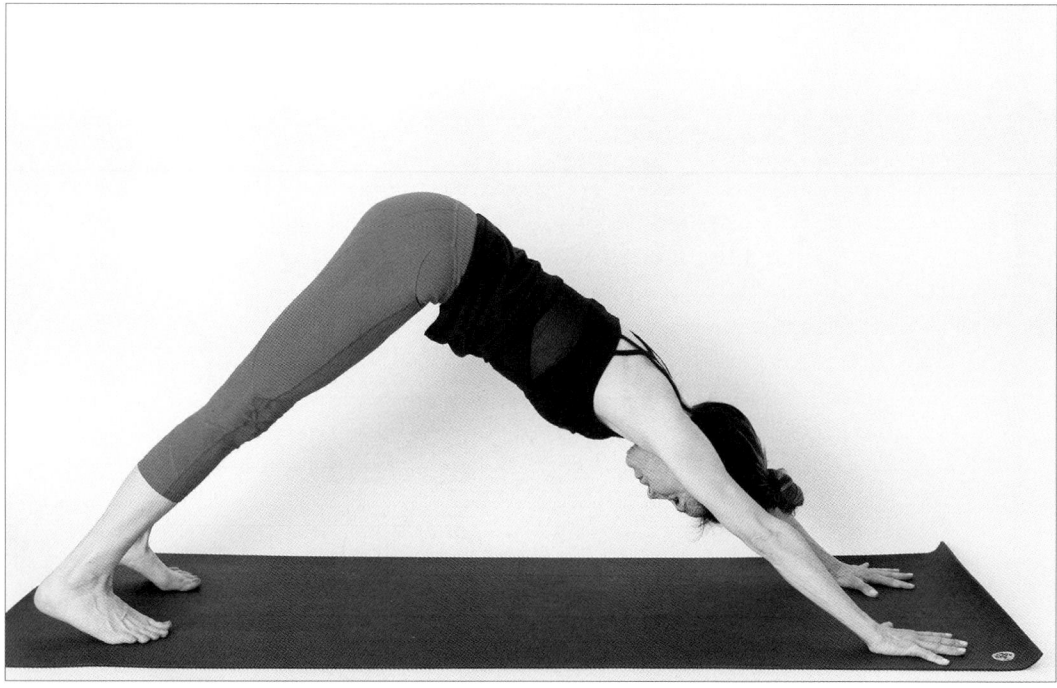

Figure 10–2.
Example of safe downward-facing dog pose

Trunk stability is even more important for firefighters because the work they do means their bodies are often out of alignment. They must continually compensate for performing frequent bending, lifting, twisting, carrying, and reaching movements while wearing gear that weighs 60 pounds or more and carrying heavy equipment. This problem is magnified for women and smaller-stature firefighters because the gear is all the same size. A number of firefighters have told me that they can now feel when their body is out of alignment after they take their gear off, so they do a few quick exercises to feel that trunk stability again. Check out the sidebar for a couple of easy exercises you can do at the station.

Quick Exercises to Realign

Lie down on your back. Extend your legs and flex your toes toward your shins. Extend your arms overhead, as if for a morning stretch. Take a couple of deep breaths while stretching your entire body. Next, bend both knees and place your palms on your thighs just below your knees. Pick up your feet and press your knees into your hands and your hands into your knees. Resisting the forward movement of your knees with the strength of your hands will activate the core and reset the pelvis. Set your feet back down and allow your knees to twist to the left while turning your head to the right. (Again, use caution and consult a doctor before attempting this if you have neck pain or a neck injury.) Hold this pose for a couple of breaths, then switch sides. This simple twist helps to align the spine.

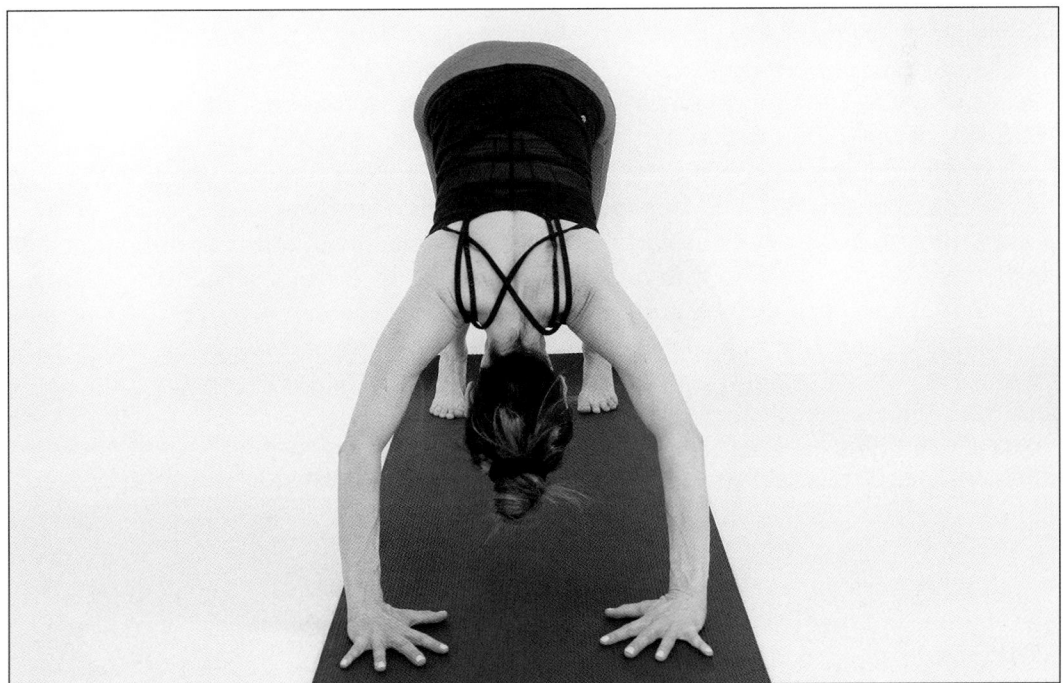

Figure 10–3.
Example of unsafe downward-facing dog pose

Going from Zero to Sixty and Back: Ujjayi Warrior Breathing

One of the best barometers I know for working with the will in a sustainable and conscious way is the breath. Staying connected to our breath allows us to work along the edge of our practice, exploring the realm just beyond our comfort zone. Finding this edge in our practice between the known and unknown is what makes yoga so interesting and keeps the practice forever fresh and dynamic. Being conscious of our breath is also what alerts us to what's happening in our bodies so we can modulate a pose to prevent injury. This interoceptive awareness translates off the mat as well because the key to steadiness and ease in the middle of overwhelming emotions is the breath.

I recently met with several fitness coordinators from the California Department of Forestry and Fire Protection (Cal Fire) to talk about training programs. I wasn't surprised when I kept hearing, "When you work with firefighters, the classes are a lot harder, right?" Because I've encountered so many assumptions about yoga, I understand that until firefighters start practicing yoga themselves, they don't get how difficult a seemingly simple pose like downward-facing dog can be. When we add practices like ujjayi breathing and guided meditations or visualizations, firefighters are amazed at how challenging it is for them to focus their attention for even a single breath.

Ujjayi breathing, sometimes called the victorious or warrior breath, is an ancient yoga practice that calms our nerves and helps us to access the courage to be with strong sensations without having to distract ourselves by tuning them out or being numb to them. The idea is to make your breath sound like waves coming up on the shore or the wind blowing through the trees. To make this sound, you'll need to constrict, or tighten, the muscles in the back of your throat as you inhale and exhale.

Humorously, ujjayi is often called Darth Vader breath. By classes 5 and 6, firefighters are beginning to feel comfortable using the breath as a tool, so even though they might feel a bit strange sounding like Darth Vader, they're willing to give it a try.

To perform ujjayi, start sitting up with a cushion or other support under your hips so that your hips are higher than your knees. Let your pelvis gently move towards your lower back, while still maintaining its natural curve. Using diaphragmatic breathing (see chapter 8), take a deep breath into your nose, gently tightening the back of your throat. Exhale with your mouth open and imagine you're fogging up the lenses of your glasses, making an extended "haah" sound. Repeat that a few times, noting that the sound is made in the back of your throat. Now, take another breath and make the fogging exhalation sound with your lips closed. Repeat for several rounds.

The breath reflects what's going on with us and how we're feeling, in both body and mind. Therefore, shallow or uneven breathing often indicates that we're feeling nervous, or even depressed. When in fight-or-flight mode, your heart starts pounding and your breath becomes rapid. Still, breath is one thing we do have control over. You can use ujjayi breathing on the mat or off to give yourself an energy boost, increase your concentration, and change your mood. The next time you're feeling stressed or uneasy, practice ujjayi for a few minutes to calm both your body and your mind.

Conclusion

Firefighters go from a dead sleep to dressed in turnouts and heading out of the station in two minutes or less. They get conditioned to using their will to get through another call, another crisis, another hour. They get used to living in overdrive.

As pointed out in chapter 4, elevated heart rates and overall stress levels don't subside when the shift ends. On the yoga mat, firefighters use this conditioned response to try and will their way through the more challenging poses. When they can't do it, they're confronted with the shadow side of the warrior culture that says, "you're a failure," or "you need to succeed," and dictates that success and victory mean pushing through no matter the cost.

On the mat, however, by consciously using your breath to stay with the poses, you can begin increasing your capacity to manage stress and remain connected to your body even in the face of difficult inner conversations with your shadow side. The reward for persevering with this new way of doing things is more self-awareness—and relief for your aching back!

11

Balancing Your Life

CLASSES 7 AND 8

Daily Movement: Developing balance for climbing ladders and stairs, stepping in and out of the rig, and working on a roof.

Functional Fitness Objective: In-line lunge

Interoceptive Awareness: Feeling the through line from the ground under your feet to the top of the head

Yoga Poses: Bridge, tree, crescent lunge

Mindfulness/Meditation: Alternate-nostril breathing

Shannon Learns Skate Skiing—Kind of

I was on vacation recently at a winter resort and decided to sign up for a one-on-one class in skate skiing. The instructor, Rick, talked to me before we started to get an idea of my experience level. Rick was a big, no-nonsense older guy who used to operate a jackhammer. I assured him that he had nothing to worry about because even though I had no experience skate skiing, I had done a lot of downhill skiing years before, and my balance was excellent from practicing and teaching yoga for 20 years. I was feeling confident and, in reflection, puffed up about how good I was going to be at this new sport.

At the flat surface where the class starts, I put on these really short, slippery, very thin skis. From downhill skiing I knew that skis are designed to be frictionless so they can glide on top of the snow, but I hadn't realized how badly these new skis were going to mess up my balance. That was the first sign that I was way out of my comfort zone.

Early on, Rick did what any good yoga instructor does when they see their students struggling—shift to plan B. Except in my case he had to go straight to plan C! He thought I was going to be a natural because that's what I told him to expect, but then he realized, "She's really awful!" He waited until after class to tell me this.

Plan C was going back to the very beginning instructions. First, practice getting balanced and stable on your skis. Then begin to walk up the hill. No poles at this point because I had to learn how to work my lower body first. Rick led and I tried to follow. Slowly. Then I led and he followed. We did this for an hour. In the beginning, I fell really hard, but my training kicked in and I bounced back up. I could see Rick nod his head in acknowledgment. Then I toppled over again. I had forgotten just how hard packed snow is: it is like hitting cement.

By this point, the flood of self-doubt and embarrassing thoughts were churning away: "Wow, you're getting old!" "I thought I was going to be good at this!" "I'm going to get hurt!" Because of my regular yoga practice, I pretty quickly became aware of what was happening, and rather than identifying too much with these deflating thoughts or being taken over by them, I was able to bring myself back into the moment. I made a few jokes about falling on my butt. Rick responded with humor of his own, which gave me time to decide I was just not going to take myself too seriously. I reminded myself that whether or not I was good at skate skiing was not going to fundamentally change who I am, and I could decide to get back into the lesson and be okay with it.

I ended up having a lot of fun, and Rick was impressed by how much I had improved by the end of the lesson. The whole experience was a powerful reminder of why I changed my life to teach yoga to first responders and the central questions that motivate me: How do we react when life doesn't show up the way we thought? How do we cope when responding to emergencies and catastrophes is a lot more demoralizing than we expected? How do we deal with not being good at something, or simply being outside our comfort zone? In the case of skate skiing, the issue was my lack of balance and my bruised ego, which was much more painful than my bruised butt.

When Getting Out of Balance Means Winning

Balancing poses seem to be particularly difficult for firefighters who don't surf, snowboard, skateboard, or skate ski—all of which require both trunk stability and balancing with the feet often in an asymmetric stance. Added to the difficulty factor is the awkwardness they feel (and not just firefighters I might add) when they fall out. Picture two rows of firefighters standing on their mats attempting a tree pose, struggling to maintain their balance, bodies rocking side to side, teeth clenched, holding their breath, and when they fall out trying to pretend it's no big deal. But there's no way to hide in these standing balance poses, as I experienced in my lesson on the ski hill.

So I ask the question: Is it worth it to feel a bit ridiculous trying to look like a tree? The answer is a resounding yes, especially when you look at some of the benefits of good balance, such as better reaction time, body awareness, coordination, and joint strength. Practicing balance poses develops the cerebellum, the part of our brain that regulates balance and coordinated movement. When firefighters tell me about the calls when they have to work on a roof while wearing heavy gear and operating a chainsaw, I remind them how a well-developed balance and coordination system comes in handy.

When you practice balance poses with a focus on interoception and mindfulness, you're building not just physical balance but also the kind of self-awareness that can lead to better situational awareness and decision-making, off the mat as well as on.

How does balance work? Think about it in terms of the big picture. In physics, two forces that are of equal magnitude and acting in opposite directions balance each other. In our nervous system, we have a similar push-pull where the body is always drawn toward homeostasis (see chapter 4 for more detail about how this yin-yang opposition works to keep our bodies in balance). What most of us don't understand until we actually study the physiologic process is that getting out of balance is how we humans adapt and grow.

Remember good stress? It's what helps us learn new skills, take risks, and expand our horizons. Thus, getting outside your comfort zone is often a positive move. Being balanced doesn't mean existing in a static state where everything remains the same—as nice as that might sound sometimes! *Dynamic balance* is when we fall and get back up, when we lose our temper and come back to center, or when we feel afraid and still move forward.

Mind-body integration is a dance that constantly moves toward homeostasis. The great thing about balance poses in yoga is that they demand complete concentration, which means harnessing the mind. There's no way to balance on one leg without minimizing distractions and quieting our mental chatter to focus our attention. This brings me to the subject of attention.

Situational Awareness: Paying Attention Is How to Keep All the Balls in the Air

In the situational awareness training he does in fire departments across the country, Dom Duckworth, fire captain and founder and director of the New England Center for Rescue and Emergency Medicine, says that "peripheral vision, distraction, and stress impact perception of change in an environment."[1] In other words, what we see isn't always as sharp or accurate as it needs to be. In crisis situations, this can lead to serious errors. The good news, according to Captain Duckworth, is that because we know the "limitations of cognition, especially when compromised by stress, failures in situational awareness are predictable." This means we know what to fix. But how?

Neuroscientist Amishi Jha brings 15 years of research into the problem of how first responders can develop better perception in high-stakes environments. Her answer? Mindfulness training. Jha studies what she calls the brain's *attention system*—that is, how the brain has evolved to deal with the 10 megabytes of information it receives every second. She explains that attention allows us to notice, select, and direct the brain's resources. She calls attention "the brain's boss" because "wherever attention goes, the rest of the brain follows."[2] Jha says that within 170 milliseconds, our perception of a particular scene changes. What stands out to each of us depends on what we pay attention to. Stress and mind wandering are the two factors that most consistently diminish our powers of perception. Just how important is even a small reduction in our powers of perception?

A friend who came back from a structure fire gave me a great description of how challenging it can be to focus. As he was taking in the information being reported by the dispatcher as well as radio traffic from other units, he was looking in the direction of the call and reading the smoke to figure out the intensity and nature of the fire. Will his crew be first, second, or third unit on scene? While all this is going on, the crew discusses plans on their headsets. As they pull on scene, they immediately take in the visible smoke and flames, the construction of the house and roof, reports from neighbors on the location of trapped persons, and the location of electrical wires and hydrants.

By this point in my friend's story, I was overwhelmed just listening. All this information has to be processed and decisions made on the best response: Do they grab a hose line or a ladder? Do they go in the front door or a side window? The point he made so powerfully is that an incredible amount of information needs to be processed by the brain almost instantaneously—and when lives are involved, the pressure on the decision maker goes up exponentially.

For more than 10 years, Jha has been doing mindfulness training with first responders and the military, usually right before or during high-stress situations—for example, just before troops deploy. She reports that when soldiers were tested two months after a training session, the control group showed that attention had gone way down while the mindfulness group stayed stable. Most exciting, those who committed to doing mindfulness exercises every day showed significant improvements in attention.

As a first responder, what are some of the benefits you could experience from practicing mindfulness? Jha says that in high-stakes environments, mindfulness could enable you to be more discerning, more present, not as reactive to fear and anxiety, and a better decision maker (refer back to "How Mindfulness Works" in chapter 3 for a refresher).

Kick-Ass Glutes?

Before we get into the balance postures, a few words about the glutes. Most of us don't think much about our posteriors except for how they look: Saggy? Flabby? Epic? Humor aside, the glutes are one of the most important muscle groups for balance, yet they are neglected by most of us, even many top athletes. The gluteus muscles—gluteus maximus, medius, and minimus—pretty much do the heavy lifting that allow our legs to do their duty. For firefighters, that includes getting up from a squatting position safely and easily, having the power needed to sprint, getting in and out of rigs, and climbing ladders. Doing balance poses is one way to find out if you have issues with your glutes. Surprisingly, plantar fasciitis often indicates that the glutes may be too weak.[3]

Common problems with the gluteus muscles include weak glutes from a lot of sitting and overdeveloped, tight glutes from overuse, particularly running on treadmills and doing deadlifts, front squats, and lunges. For firefighters, weak glutes are common. The first sign may be low scores on the squatting exercise on the FMS or the pelvis tilting to one side when a firefighter tries to balance on one leg. Weak glutes and tight IT bands (the IT bands are connective tissues that run along the outside of your legs from the top of the pelvis to the shins) can lead to back, hip, knee, and pelvic pain, as well as poor posture.

Compounding the problem of weak glutes, we often compensate by using our hip flexors to give us the strength we need to complete a movement. The hip flexors are the muscles near the top of your thighs that let you walk, kick, bend, and swivel your hips. However, compensating with weak or tight hip flexors will merely exacerbate lower back and hip pain and increase the chances of injury over time.[4]

In the poses described in this chapter, I give modifications that will let you make necessary adjustments as you build up your glute and hip flexor stability. You can also go back to the poses in classes 1 and 2 to help with mobility and stability in your hips.

Poses: Bridge, Tree, and Crescent Lunge

Extensive research has shown that physical exercise changes the brain in ways that improve our thinking. Balancing exercises in particular show changes in the areas of the brain that control memory and spatial cognition. This is neuroplasticity in action![5] To best engage the brain's ability to create new neural patterns, we need to practice balancing in one position and then make it more challenging by adding movement. Therefore, this sequence goes from static to more dynamic poses.

Bridge

I often use bridge as an anticipatory pose to activate and strengthen the glutes. It's lower risk because firefighters are resting most of their body weight on the floor.

To do bridge, begin by lying on your back, with your knees bent. Feet should be about a hip-width apart and parallel, with your heels in line with the sitting bones, your upper back resting on the mat, and your hands by your hips with palms down. Remember to find your neutral pelvis position. As you exhale, lift the hips lift away from the mat, and on inhalation, lower the hips back down. As you lift, gently tuck the pelvis under just before lifting the hips; this action prevents overarching (hyperextending) the lower back. Gently lift the upper back and draw the shoulder blades closer together to open the front of the body; this will stretch the internal rotators of the shoulders and chest muscles. Repeat the lifting and lowering movements a few times, in concert with your breath. On the final round, hold your hips level for four to six breaths before lowering your hips to the mat.

Firefighters with weak glutes and tight hip flexors tend to turn their toes outward to get more leverage to lift their hips. Also, weak glutes and tight hip flexors will prevent the hips from lifting very high. One modification of bridge is to put your feet on blocks. This will allow your hips to move into the pose more easily.

Tree

There are so many ways to do a tree pose. My preference for firefighters is to start with a version where they feel the external rotation in their hips prior to balancing. This pose strengthens the leg muscles, ankles, feet, and hips while stabilizing the trunk, especially hips and spine.

Begin with feet hip-width apart, standing tall and making sure your ankles, hips, and shoulders are aligned. Shift your weight to your right leg and bring your left foot onto the inside of your right calf. Your toes should still be touching the floor while your left heel is lifted onto the inner right shin. Focus your gaze either on a point in front of you at eye level or on the floor. Pick something to focus on that is not moving. Find your breath and keep it moving even and steady; then, when you're ready, begin slowly sliding your left foot up the inner right shin to either just below the knee or just above it if you can. You are now balancing on one leg. Hands can be on your hips or palms pressing together at the chest. Slowly lower your left foot to the floor and switch sides.

Wobbling and falling out of this pose are common challenges. If your hip dips toward the standing leg, that will cause your pelvis to be no longer level, or neutral. One modification is to keep the toes of your left foot on the ground while you work on externally rotating your left hip and stabilizing the standing leg, keeping the pelvis level. Shallow, strained breathing is a giveaway of overexertion going on, so remember to keep your breath smooth and steady.

Crescent lunge

Even though this is a challenging pose, by this class, firefighters are more grounded and have a better sense of who they are on the mat. We've shared laughter and had fun as they've gradually built up the inner strength needed for these later classes. They feel more comfortable taking charge of their own practice, so I feel comfortable giving directions and then getting out of the way.

Start in mountain pose (see chapter 9) with feet hip-width apart. Take a long step back with your left foot and pivot onto the ball of that foot. The front foot is flat (without collapsing the arch). Both feet should be pointing toward the front of the mat yet remain hip-width apart. Begin to bend the front leg while straightening the back leg. If by straightening the back leg, you move your front knee past the front ankle, then increase your stance (the distance between front and back legs). Keep the front of your pelvis lifting away from the front thigh, which activates the core. Reach your fingertips toward the mat, rotate your thumbs away, externally rotating through your arms and shoulders, and then lift both arms overhead. Slowly bend and lower the back knee toward the mat, and then lift and straighten. Do this a few times before holding the pose with a straight back leg.

Refine the pose with the following steps. Press down through both feet and lift the trunk, so that it is vertical and perpendicular to the floor, and then extend through the spine. Keep lifting the front of the pelvis away from the front thigh while extending the tailbone toward the mat. With arms overhead, relax (soften) at the tops of the shoulders to increase space between shoulders and ears (trapezius). Lift the waist out of the pelvis to lengthen the side body. Remember to breathe!

The main challenge in crescent lunge is keeping your balance. If you're having trouble, keep your back leg bent or put your knee on the floor. The tip from the tree pose also applies here: to help you balance, focus on a spot in front of you.

Alternate-Nostril Breathing

There are good reasons so many firefighters come to rely on the breathing techniques they learn in yoga classes to help them manage stress. One highly effective technique, *alternate-nostril breathing*, is particularly good for attaining balance. Yes, I know the name is weird, and doing it might feel a bit strange at first; however, I think you'll find it well worth the effort.

This technique works by balancing the right and left hemispheres of the brain. In a review article, Dr. Shreya Ghiya found that across 44 randomized controlled trials, "This technique provides high level evidence for positive outcomes for the autonomic nervous and cardiopulmonary systems. There is also high level of evidence regarding improvement in cognitive functioning."[6]

So get your nostrils ready! Below are the steps to perform alternate-nostril breathing:

1. Rest your left palm on your left knee, and bring your right hand toward your nose.
2. Take a deep breath, and when you exhale take your right thumb and gently close your right nostril.
3. Inhale slowly through the left nostril, then close it with the ring finger of your right hand. Both nostrils will now be closed. Hold the breath for a moment.
4. Take your thumb away from the right nostril and exhale slowly. Hold the breath on the exhale for a moment.
5. Inhale slowly through the right nostril, then close it with the thumb. Pause.
6. Open the left nostril and exhale slowly. Then inhale through the left and close the nostril.
7. Open the right nostril and exhale.
8. Repeat this pattern five to ten times, and then gently bring your breathing back to normal.

Thus, the basic pattern is inhale left, exhale right, inhale right, exhale left, repeat.

If you have a cold or your nasal passages are clogged you might want to wait to do this. Also, if you have high blood pressure, check with your doctor before trying this.

Conclusion

I credit yoga with learning that surrender doesn't have to mean losing, at least not losing in the way the traditional warrior culture thinks about it. Balance sequences, especially once you get to more challenging ones like sun salutation, can make you face your limitations head on.

Yoga poses can be incredibly frustrating, disorienting, and even defeating. The question I ask is: What would happen if you could let your guard down, even 5%, while you struggle with a pose? Rather than feeling like you're failing, experience what surrendering to the moment feels like. What new knowledge or information might show up to help you to solve the problem? Try making a minor adjustment, or perhaps you've been forgetting to breathe (happens all the time); you may need to drop out of the pose for a minute to regroup, then come back ready for another attempt.

Yoga can teach us the habit of making micro adjustments on the fly. While our attention still wanders, we learn to bring it back in a moment. This kind of self-awareness can lead to living a balanced life with the skills to better navigate both the demands of work and family and the uncertainty that comes with the job. Better self-awareness leads to enhanced situational awareness and greater self-regulation. Ultimately, this can be lifesaving for the public as well as for first responders.

12

#ItAllConnects

CLASSES 9–10

Daily Movement: Connecting mobility and stability for getting up and down from the floor or chair, lifting, squatting, and lunging

Functional Fitness Objective: Deep squat

Interoceptive Awareness: Feeling deep flexion in ankles, knees, and hips

Yoga Poses: Toe squat, happy baby, cobbler's

Mindfulness/Meditation: Loving kindness (metta)

Systems Thinking: Resilience through Yoga—for Corporate Boardrooms and Fire Stations

When Tony Schwartz and Jim Loehr work with executives on performance improvement, they take a holistic approach based on Loehr's 20 years of coaching top athletes. In their hugely popular articles and books, they emphasize that sustained high performance—managing a high-stress career over the long term—requires attention to our whole self: body, emotions, mind, and spirit. They also warn that performance is compromised when we fail to deal with any one of these dimensions.[1]

Schwartz and Loehr are using the *systems thinking* approach. This same theory is represented in the mind-body-spirit foundation of yoga. I'm thrilled that a yogic, holistic approach is used in settings like corporate boardrooms and sports arenas and delighted that these authors include spirit and emotions in their system, which are so often neglected in performance training. The touchy-feely stuff is particularly tough to talk about in first responder groups. Nevertheless, it's imperative that we do. The bottom line is that the systems approach is about resilience—both physical and mental. You can't bounce back from stressful situations, especially not at full capacity, if one part of the system is down.

When Schwartz and Loehr talk about spirit, they mean deeper values and a sense of purpose. It's human nature to look for a sense of purpose to give meaning to our lives, and when I talk about spirit in yoga, I don't mean from a strictly religious perspective. Instead, yoga and meditation practices clear emotional and psychological clutter so we can more clearly experience what our mind-body system is telling us, bringing us closer to what truly motivates us.

Everything Is Just Fine

Emotions and feelings can be intimidating to talk about, particularly for anyone who lacks skills to process emotions. But after personally examining many painful emotions in my own body, I've gotten pretty fearless! Until we experience emotions as sensations in the body (interoception) and learn to name them, we can't do anything to change them—or, in the case of an emotion like love, even fully enjoy them. Because of the negativity bias humans are hardwired to have (see chapter 3), it's easy to get stuck in an endless loop of depression, anxiety, negative thoughts, or victim consciousness, often leading to a closed mindset where we feel there's nothing we can do—in other words, we feel as though we have no agency.

A big challenge for firefighters is that much of the stress they face comes from battling what society doesn't want to deal with—namely, rampant homelessness, catastrophic medical emergencies such as mass-casualty incidents, and an opioid epidemic. This is ugly stuff. The first responders I work with recall way too many mind-numbing encounters with squalor and hopelessness, often feeling that there is nothing they can do to change anything. Add to this being chronically overworked and not being able to sleep at night because of what they see. Frank Leto, deputy director of counseling unit in the FDNY, says that firefighting is a career of accumulation.[2]

One of the statements I often hear from first responders is, "This is not what I signed up for and spent years training to do." I hear their growing demoralization and try to help with their burnout. These are some of the questions circling around the firehouses I work in: How do you retain your humanity and not get jaded? How do you return home every day after what you've seen and be a parent and relate to the other people in your life? Jeff Dill (founder and director of the Firefighter Behavioral Health Alliance), who I've mentioned several times in the book, is concerned about how bitter many firefighters become and how no one is talking about it.

What I find so amazing and inspires me to keep going is the dedication and commitment of the firefighters I work with. Day after day they show up no matter the cost to themselves. What I see is that when shown ways to increase resilience that make sense and actually work, they're all in. Through a single yoga class, firefighters receive the benefits and understand the need.

This chapter is about how yoga and mindfulness promote resilience for firefighters by helping them develop a relationship with their bodies. This physical resilience becomes their first level of support, the canary in the coal mine so to speak. Because if you can listen to what your body is telling you, you can do something about it.

Safety Cues versus Danger Cues

A couple of years ago, I was presenting the benefits of yoga to a group of decision makers for a fire department. Part of my presentation deals with the aspects of acute and long-term stress, including post-traumatic stress (injury or both disorder and injury). After describing how trauma lives in the body and nervous system, I noticed patterns among the most common reactions people had:

- Wanting an unawareness of their body because it's too painful
- Staying in a constant state of hypervigilance
- Feeling numb, like they don't even have a body
- Being unaware of signals to stop overeating, drinking alcohol to excess, or engaging in other risky behavior

Yet they can't talk about what's happening because they don't have the words. The department captain, who had been listening intently throughout my presentation, suddenly started talking. "I think that's me," he said, sounding a little shocked. "When I get off work, the only way I can feel like myself again is to take my mountain bike to the top of a mountain and head straight down, no brakes. Then I feel something, my heart racing, the adrenaline rush." It was an intense moment when he started realizing what the accumulation of chronic stress was leading him to do.

What was happening while the captain was riding his bike down the mountain? Neuroscientist Steven Porges says that extreme sports and exercise and other risky behaviors can sometimes be an attempt to avoid shutting down all feelings entirely. Porges explains that our nervous system has evolved two responses to threat or danger: either we go into fight-or-flight mode or, if we feel there's no way out of a situation, we try to immobilize—basically shut down or go numb. However, our nervous system knows that totally shutting down is not physiologically acceptable, so feeling danger and the rush of adrenaline lets us feel something while we suppress other emotions we think we can't handle.[3]

In people who experience trauma or long-term stress, the nervous system continues to perceive danger cues in the environment long after the inciting event. Even being asked to communicate our feelings (by a spouse or partner, for example) can be a danger cue if emotions are suppressed because they're too frightening to experience. The most important thing we can do, according to Porges, is to learn to differentiate between safety cues and danger cues, then turn off the threat cues when appropriate so that we can feel safe enough to engage fully in our lives.[4] Therefore, we must ask how the body can become our ally in this process.

Interoceptive Yoga: Building Resilience through Awareness

Here's a recap of how interoception works. Emotions, including the most intense (anger, fear, and love), come from the complex and continuous communication loop between the body and brain. The body sends signals to the brain about our outer and inner environment: Is there a threat coming from the outside? Is my gut telling me something isn't right? Am I feeling comfortable and safe? By the time we recognize these feelings or emotions, the brain has already received the signals from the body and sent back messages. If you are reading the signals correctly, there are windows of opportunity when you can decide what to do.

I was working with an EMT the other day and she told me that, while she learned about recovery in the academy, it was only in practicing yoga that she finally understood how to do it. Before yoga, she was experiencing one adrenaline dump after the other and starting to burn out. Now, on the way to a call, she checks in with her body and uses breathing practices to stay connected. By being present, she said, she was regulating her energy, and it had become a positive habit. Managing our energy is one excellent way to manage the tricky art of work-life balance.

Putting this down in writing makes it sound easy. In no way do I mean to imply that doing yoga or meditation, or just becoming aware of signals from your body, is a quick fix to manage intense emotions. However, after working with firefighters for many years, I see that yoga and mindfulness practices do serve as valuable tools for achieving long-term psychological resilience.

In chapter 10, I told the story of recovering from a serious motorcycle accident, particularly the idea of gradual microrecoveries over time. One of the most powerful results from the early days of my recovery is how yoga helped me to be in my body, to be relaxed and still—a new reference point for how to be. I hadn't even realized how stressed I was, but I finally found myself allowing feelings like joy to arise again. Through not allowing myself to feel uncomfortable emotions like stress, I was also not allowing myself to feel pleasurable emotions. Yoga had let me define a new normal. Not that I feel joy all the time—I wish! I'm certainly not smiling all the time, nor is that what resilience requires.

Interoceptive yoga works so well for first responders because it's a unique method of relating to and working with the body. Exercise and the feel-good cocktail of hormones it releases—endorphins, endocannabinoids, and dopamine—boosts optimism as well as reduces tension in the body.[5]

Most of the firefighters I work with are brand-new to yoga, but those who have already taken a class or two described the style of yoga that they gravitated toward (not surprisingly) as similar to boot camp—a teacher yelling orders while loud rock music pumps through the steamy, humid air. Not that this style isn't fun sometimes—I enjoy lifting weights and taking an occasional hot yoga class when I need a serious sweat—but in a culture that constantly tells us to do more, produce more, create more, be more, it's dangerously easy to make exercise, even yoga, an arena for pushing your body to the extreme. By contrast, interoceptive yoga focuses more on self-awareness. Interoceptive yoga slows down the practice, requiring more time in the poses, leading to increased awareness of both body and mind. Along with conscious control of the breath and mindfulness exercises, interoceptive yoga teaches us how to balance high intensity with ease and how to cycle between effort and relaxation—exactly as our central nervous system is built to balance stress and recovery. Practicing opens up our mindset, creating the space to make better, healthier choices, including knowing when to seek outside help. It's trusting our bodies so we can trust ourselves.

Poses: Toe Squat, Happy Baby, and Cobbler's

This sequence requires the flexibility and strength developed from practicing all the poses in the previous eight weeks of the program: a stable trunk; ankle, knee, and hip flexion and mobility; and strong gluteal and flexible leg muscles. As preliminary poses, these three develop lower body mobility and strength and eventually lead to performing the deep squat well.

The deep squat is the first exercise in the FMS, so it is the first one I do with firefighters in my program. It might seem counterintuitive to start the FMS with an exercise that's challenging to do correctly, but the deep squat is an excellent overall baseline.

Usually, firefighters can do a deep squat when they turn out their feet. However, the intent of the FMS is to bring to the surface how we *compensate* for certain weaknesses. Therefore, the FMS has people do the squat with feet parallel and shoulder width apart; firefighters typically are not initially able to do this successfully. Turning the feet out is a way to compensate for weak or tight hips. Furthermore, I often see heels lifting off the floor to get hips lower while still keeping the trunk vertical and shoulders in full flexion with a dowel hanging overhead (see fig. 6–1 for an image of the deep squat). This compensation signals, among other things, a lack of ankle mobility. With the FMS's guidance, if I see firefighters lifting their heels, I have them put their heels on a board and repeat the movement three times. If this assistance makes it easier for them to lower their hips, then this becomes a safe starting point for poses that stretch the feet and increase ankle mobility.

Connective tissue: holding it all together

Connective tissue comprises our tendons, ligaments, and fascia. Fascia is the shrink-wrap material that surrounds and connects all the joints, muscles, and organs in our body. It's mostly made up of *collagen*, the stretchy material that is sometimes called the glue that holds the body together.

Yin yoga, which focuses exclusively on connective tissues, is growing in popularity. Some firefighters tell me they do only yin yoga because they see it as a deeper, slower practice that targets the body in a way that other styles don't. By contrast, *yang* yoga (active), as with most exercise, focuses on the muscles (yang tissues).

Classes 9 and 10 include fast-moving, more intense poses that stress muscle issues over a shorter period of time. Depending on the group, I might also incorporate more intensity through a yin approach. Yin applies a gentle steady force that brings moisture, oxygen, and other biological resources to the yin tissues or fascia. This practice coaxes the fascia into becoming stronger and supports joint mobility. Again, depending on the group, I might have firefighters hold a pose for only a single breath or up to a few minutes.

Therapeutic ball warm-up

Using therapeutic balls is a terrific way to prepare for any yoga practice. To warm up the fascia before exercise or yoga, start with the feet. To try this warm-up, grab a small firm ball—such as a tennis ball, lacrosse ball, or a therapy ball. Start standing up, and place the ball under the widest part of one foot. Wrap the ball with your toes, like a bird on a perch. Squeeze and release, twice in a row. Then move the ball to the middle of the foot and roll it around the whole middle of your foot, between pads of your toes and heel. Last, put the ball right under your heel, then press down and release. Repeat this a few times. This is such a terrific warm-up that if you try to touch your toes afterward, you'll be surprised at how much more agile you are.

Toe squat

This pose stretches the fascia of the feet, toes, and ankles. Begin on your hands and knees in tabletop. Draw your knees and inner ankles closer together. Tuck your toes and sit back on your heels. Stay in the pose as long as you can keep your breath steady and even. Come out of the pose by leaning forward onto your hands and gently tapping the tops of your feet into the mat. The most common challenge is toes that won't flex at all, like pieces of wood. If this happens to you, try the following modifications:

- Keep your fingertips on the floor to avoid bearing all your weight on your toes
- Place both knees on a folded blanket or bolster to reduce the pressure on the soles of your feet and on the toes

Happy baby

This is an inverted deep squat that builds ankle, knee, and hip flexion. Start on your back with knees bent. Draw both knees toward your chest. Reach out and grab hold of either the inner or outer aspect of both feet. Use your arms to open your feet and draw your knees toward your armpits. Point the soles of your feet toward the ceiling and flex your toes toward your shins as if you could stand on the ceiling. Draw your tailbone toward the mat. To release, let go of your feet and place them back on the mat, hip-width apart.

Yes, this pose looks as ridiculous as it sounds! Fortunately, by this point in the program, firefighters are used to laughing together as a group activity and usually crack up as they tackle looking like happy babies. Their enjoyment and the willingness to be vulnerable is a great indication that the program has been a success.

Modifications include:

- Grabbing hold of your ankles or shins, if you can't reach your feet
- Placing a strap around the balls of both feet
- Bringing up one let at a time, if you can't bring both legs up

Cobbler's

This pose requires flexion and external rotation in hips, flexion in ankles and knees, and flexibility in inner legs. This is necessary for knees to release toward the floor and the hip to descend deeply.

Seated, draw your legs out in front of you so that your torso and thighs form an angle (ideally 90°). Bend your knees and draw the soles of your feet together toward the groin, paying attention to your knees as you draw your heels as close as you comfortably can toward your groin. Gently press your knees toward the floor. Interlace your fingers around your toes and the outer edges of your feet. Draw your torso up and lengthen your spine before folding forward.

For some, the challenge is sitting upright on the floor. Modifications include:

- Laying on your back, drawing the soles of your feet together, and letting your knees drop down toward the floor
- Sliding blocks underneath your knees to prevent overstretching of your inner thighs

Mindfulness for Better Performance and Less Burnout

In their article "Role of Resilience in Mindfulness Training for First Responders," psychologist Josh Kaplan and colleagues studied law enforcement officers and firefighters who completed an eight-week Mindfulness-Based Stress Reduction training program. Their results showed that "increased mindfulness was related to increased resilience, which in turn was related to decreased burnout."[6] What I find really exciting about the mindfulness research being done, including this study, is that *nonreactivity* is increased. This doesn't mean becoming like a zombie. It means having more control over how we react to what's happening and being better able to manage our feelings, whether they be frustration, anger, or sadness.

An increased ability to focus in intense situations is another benefit of mindfulness. This is why meditation has become so popular with elite athletes. One proponent of mindfulness in sports is George Mumford, the renowned meditation coach of stars such as Michael Jordan and Kobe Bryant. In an interview with ABC News, Munford said practicing mindfulness helps his clients get in the zone. "If you really look at the elite athletes, you will find they have this ability to be in a moment and actually slow things down," he told ABC News. "When a basketball player is caught thinking about the shot they just missed, they are more likely to miss the shot in the next moment. Meditation techniques help people to train their minds to stay in the present without getting caught up thinking about other stressors."[7]

Loving Kindness

This form of meditation, also called metta, expands to encompass everyone and everything. Loving kindness has been shown to have numerous benefits—from helping cope with chronic pain, to higher-level perspective taking and emotion regulation.[8] So why not try this one?

To practice metta, pick three or four phrases, also referred to as *affirmations*, that are significant to you. Then repeat them, starting with yourself and moving to other people in your life. You start with yourself because you are as worthy of loving kindness as anyone else. The reason is that to care for and help others, you must first care for yourself (this is the same as when you're flying: you would put on your own oxygen mask before you put on your child's).

When my friend, Division Chief David Dolson, teaches metta in his station, he explains that as first responders you can only give what you have to give, so if you're feeling low you have to replenish your own reserves. I've learned to do this meditation using a series of different phrases. The following four are commonly used: may I be happy, may I be healthy, may I be safe, and may I experience peace. You can change the phrases to fit what's happening in your life at the moment.

Find a comfortable place to perform this, either seated or lying down. Close your eyes if you want. Repeat the above phrases starting with yourself, aloud or silently in your head. Then move on to someone you love, and as you picture them, repeat the phrases a few times: may you be happy, may you be healthy, may you be safe, may you experience peace. Then move to a neutral person, someone you might see at the grocery store or walking their dog in the neighborhood but don't have a relationship with, and repeat the phrases. Next, move to a difficult person, someone who challenges you, and repeat the phrases. Don't worry if this is difficult or brings up negative feelings, just keep repeating the phrase. Last, include all living things and repeat.

Conclusion

One definition of resilience that I really like is that it's getting through pain and disappointment without letting them crush your spirit. The American Psychological Association says that you're resilient if you have the following traits:

- The capacity to make realistic plans and take steps to carry them out
- A positive view of yourself and confidence in your strengths and abilities
- Skills in communication and problem solving
- The capacity to manage strong feelings and impulses[9]

Somewhere in the middle of these two definitions is where most of us live.

For first responders, being resilient is much tougher. This story from my firefighter friend, Deputy Chief Eric Vollmer, is the most inspiring and beautiful testament to the power of having good resources and the support of people who love us. Vollmer was finishing up a 10-week mindfulness training. One exercise in particular the firefighters commented on was the loving kindness meditation. Eric's daughter, who was seven years old when this story takes place, was consistently having trouble falling asleep, so every night before bed he would do some breathing exercises with her, ending with the loving kindness meditation. One night, after Eric had experienced a particularly tough day, his daughter looked at him with great love and said, "Daddy, may you be happy, may you be healthy, and may you experience peace."

Part VI

The Conscious Warrior

13

The Conscious Warrior

A MIND-BODY APPROACH TO LEADERSHIP

Leading during the Pandemic: Heroes in Hazmat Suits

In early April of 2020, Captain Dave Gillotte, with the Los Angeles County Fire Department, watched the firefighters in his station, friends he's worked with for years, get ready to respond to a medical call in the new world of the coronavirus pandemic. They gown up, goggle up, and glove up as Captain Gillotte, a union president with more than 30 years of experience, watches. He's already reviewing the protocols for monitoring where every piece of equipment will be put when they get to the scene—what's going to get touched and what isn't—and when every piece of equipment will be sanitized. He's making decisions to limit how many of his people will touch the patient: one person for the initial response, two as they move the patient, then the ambulance attendants, all while making sure everyone else keeps six feet of distance, weighing every decision to make sure everyone stays as safe as possible.

This is how Gillotte described to me what's going on in his firehouse, a scene being enacted throughout Los Angeles and the rest of the country. When I talked to him in April, he sounded remarkably composed as he described the calls his crew is going on. One was a full arrest where a COVID-19–positive person died; on another, a woman with COVID-19 symptoms gave birth. "In these kinds of medical situations, aerosoliz[ing] procedures take place," said Gillotte,, "and our level of attention to detail not only for the delivery but for our safety is in play." Because the disease spreads via droplets, any aerosol-generating medical procedure puts first responders at high risk.

"We have these grand hero moments, especially during terrible fires, where people really get to see what we do," Gillotte told me. "But the other day I was watching a young paramedic, just a few years on the job with a brand-new family at home, and he was up close and personal with a patient, trying to save his life, and it occurred to me right there that this is a hero moment. And day by day, call by call, with every firefighter, there are so many hero moments happening right now." As he explained, "Call volume is down, call intensity is up."

I hadn't planned on interviewing Gillotte about leading during the pandemic. As fate would have it, though, I was almost finished writing this chapter just as COVID-19 started its rampage through the United States. I had been talking to leaders in the fire service for months. A pandemic was not something I ever imagined I would need to address. If there's one reliable thing about being a leader, it's that you never know what's around the corner and what you're going to have to do to protect the people under your watch.

For me, the California sheltering-at-home decree meant my yoga business pretty much came to a standstill overnight. After the initial shock and disbelief, I reached for the practices and strategies I knew would help me through this difficult situation. My body had been telling me for a long time that I had been pushing myself beyond what was reasonable or healthy, so I gave myself permission to feel my exhaustion, as well as my depression and fear that the business I had spent many years building might dissolve. What would I do next? Would my brand survive? What would happen to my employees? All unanswerable questions that kept churning through my mind.

Allowing myself to feel these emotions fortunately gave me a window to see my own strength and new possibilities. I reached out to friends, I increased my yoga and exercise practice, I found more time to do short meditations and mindfulness exercises, and in sum, I worked to find a new homeostasis in the unknown.

Mostly what I did was work on opening up my mindset. I talked to departments to see what they needed and if we could move classes online; I started doing more virtual yoga programs; I worked one-on-one with some of my employees to help them file for unemployment; I spent time with my husband, taking long walks. In other words, I took care of my own mental and physical resiliency. Another way of saying this is, "I worked my own shit." Retired Lieutenant Rich Goerling, founder of the Mindful Badge Initiative, refers to this phase as the need to deal with your own trauma first.

As of mid-May 2020, when I finished writing this chapter, a lot of questions are still unanswered. What I do know is that working your own shit is the only way to the other side of trauma and fear. This is what leadership is about, and it's an ongoing process.

Although what I'm facing is tough, it's a fraction of what first responders around the world face. Again, first responders are heroes, but again the big question is, at what cost? They are heroes who are also human, with all the flaws, complexities, and challenges that come with it. This is the most important reason why I wrote this book, and repaying this debt has become even more imperative.

Most of the material in this chapter is unchanged—the prepandemic content. To this, I've added some new information, such as my conversations with Gillotte. The fact is, what good leaders do doesn't change, just the enormity of the consequences.

What Is Leadership in the New Fire Service?

"Lead me, follow me, or get out of my way." This quote, attributed to World War II General George S. Patton Jr., is the perfect slogan for the traditional warrior culture and the leadership model that has been prevalent in the fire service for generations. How applicable is it for our current generation of first responders, though?

The same quote begins Thomas Warren's insightful article in *Fire Engineering*. In the article, Warren explains that although the combat model, with its "unwavering discipline," is still necessary in today's fire service, the fact that combat mode makes up a smaller part of what firefighters do day to day means "today's fire officers need to add a new and wider dimension to their leadership skills."[1] The pandemic is only making this idea more relevant. If the combat model is not enough to thrive in today's fire service, then what is necessary in its place?

In an article for the International Association of Fire Chiefs, Battalion Chief Jo-Ann Lorber lists five core competencies for leaders:

- Leading people
- Leading change
- Communicating and building coalitions
- Exercising business judgment
- Being results driven

For leaders in the fire service, Lorber explains that "change is the most difficult competency to deal with." Given that the fire service "prefers tradition to change," the accomplishments of firefighters who are leading change in their firehouses and departments become even more outstanding.[2]

In Their Words: Firefighters Talk about What Needs to Be Done

Leadership is a huge topic and even just for the fire service remains beyond the scope of this book. Therefore, in this chapter, I focus on the area of leadership I do know best, *transformational leadership*, which deals specifically with guiding change. To narrow this down further, I describe how leadership is being implemented by the firefighters I've worked with and interviewed, specifically how they promote mind-body resiliency and an environment of openness where firefighters feel it's okay to reach out for help. These leaders have taken seriously the growing focus in the fire service on behavioral health initiatives and have led the way in their stations and departments. In other words, they are taking on the difficult challenge of being an agent of change in the development of a conscious warrior culture. Each of them has brought practices like yoga and mindfulness to their departments because they understand that firefighters need to be internally prepared, as well as tactically and operationally prepared. They understand, usually from personal experience, that self-care is not a weakness, but a strength.

This chapter includes stories and interviews from many fire captains, battalion chiefs, and department chiefs I've worked with. The sections of this chapter detail the five traits most important for change agents, no matter their leadership style or the latest leadership philosophy trending in the fire service. Each of the leaders I talked to exhibits all of these traits.

Trait 1: Having an Open Mindset

Having an open, or flexible, mindset leads to better decision-making, a mark of successful leaders. Being open to new ideas and new information and not being afraid to try different approaches to traditional ways of doing things are hallmarks of leaders who have an open mindset. Even so, not all change is good—always look at all the facts and check your bullshit detector. In the end, though, good leaders are willing to buck tradition. Most importantly, they're willing to adapt.

Critical incident stress management and peer counseling

Redding (CA) Fire Chief Cullen Kreider was filling in as interim chief in 2018, with no intention of staying on in the job and trying to fill the shoes of the predecessor he greatly admired and who was beloved by his community. He certainly had no plans on becoming a change agent in bringing behavioral health training to his department. He was just a few months into his interim position when, in his words, "all hell broke out," as what became known as the Carr Fire began its devastating rampage across his city. Basically, the whole west side of the city was on fire: more than 260 houses were destroyed, and the department lost one of their own battling the fire, Kreider recalled.

Everything changed for his department after the Carr Fire. "Prior to 2018, we didn't like to talk about our feelings, meet with counselors, open up to our chaplains, even let anyone know that we might have a weakness or were even thinking about trauma or suicide," Kreider said. "Throughout my career as a firefighter, no matter what you saw or heard or witnessed, you just sucked it up and toughed it out. We got a real slap in the face when this hit our department and our community."

Watching how much his firefighters were hurting, Kreider stepped up to help. This meant overcoming his own resistance to talking about the effects of the job. It also meant taking on the responsibilities of chief full time, one being to speak to the community about the Carr Fire over and over again—at town meetings, service-group presentations, and even in a documentary film. "It was very painful reliving the Carr Fire and the LODD [line-of-duty death]," Kreider explained.

Meditation

Research on Navy SEALs and elite adventure athletes has shown that they "have mental attributes that are also cultivated by *meditation*" [italics mine, here and below]. This and other top attributes identified apply to the leaders in the fire service.[7]

1. **In tune with their bodily sensations.** They are more likely to notice if their heart is racing or if they have tightness in a muscle. The scientific term for this state is "*interoception*" and it refers to the ability to help the brain maintain the body's natural equilibrium by bringing awareness to bodily sensations.
2. **More focused.** They spend more time in an "intentional mode," as opposed to mind wandering, the default mental state for most people. Not surprisingly, those who spend more time focused on the task at hand will likely be higher performers than those who are constantly distracted.
3. **Not averse to challenge.** Instead of fleeing or avoiding stressful situations, they orient toward difficulty and are more likely to deal well with whatever is happening around them. The scientists believe that the ability to face stressful situations head-on alleviates some of the long-term negative health effects of stress.[3]

One of the first measures Kreider took was to resurrect the long-dormant peer support group and send a team for training. As Kreider explained it, "A firefighter might not want to tell me, as their chief, that they're upset about a difficult call, but a trained peer support person can reach out with a simple, 'Hey, heard you went on a hanging today and just checking in.'"

> Ultimately the job of a leader is to empower their people. Focus on their growth and experience. Allow them space to do things their own way and give them support and validation to stay motivated and keep going.
>
> —Jenn Panko, fire captain,
> Santa Clara, CA, Fire Department

He and his team have also started regular *critical incident stress debriefings* (CISDs). After three child deaths in five days, one of which was a two-week-old whose mother was so drunk she smothered the baby in her sleep, Kreider called a CISD for everyone involved. Three fire crews, three ambulance companies, the police officers involved, chaplains, the police peer support group, and dispatchers all attended. Kreider said the feedback was positive, and people found it very helpful.

Kreider's story is particularly moving because even though he spent 30 years inside the traditional warrior culture in the fire service, he was able to change direction and see the value in doing things a new way. "The mental health part is so important," he told me. Moreover, he was honest about the challenges of managing his own stress as chief. Yoga breathing has been particularly helpful, he said, "when I take a moment to just breathe and get ready for my day." He thinks that when firefighters get introduced to yoga and meditation and experience the benefits, they will be able to create a balanced routine, one that encompasses such diverse practices as endurance training, aerobics, and yoga.

Transparency: acknowledgment from leadership

Captain Jenn Panko also serves as temporary duty chief officer at the Santa Clara City (CA) Fire Department. Panko spent almost seven years spearheading a comprehensive health and wellness program for her department. In her experience, acknowledgment by the organization's leadership of the behavioral health issues firefighters face is the single biggest factor in expediting the establishment of programs that address resiliency.

Captain Panko talked about how difficult the topic of mental health can be to discuss openly in the fire service. It has been traditionally seen as taboo, negative, embarrassing, or a weakness. Panko is excited that in the past few years, the stress firefighters deal with is finally being acknowledged and discussed more openly by the leadership. In her experience, firefighters' stress comes not only from responding to traumatic incidents, but also from everyday challenges, such as working on a 24- or 48-hour shift schedule, missing family events and holidays, and responding to the ever-changing community needs. "Now there's a system we've put in place to turn for help when you're in trouble," Panko explained.

Panko's leadership style combines tenacity with an open mindset. Her ability to see new ways of supporting resilience helped her embrace yoga and mindfulness, bringing their benefits to the new health and wellness program. Her tenacity allowed her to successfully pioneer the first fitness program based on yoga techniques in the department. "Fitness is holistic," Panko told me, "and programs like yours that promote both physical fitness through functional movement and a psychological safe space to focus on mental health are critical in this line of work. Especially helpful are the breathing techniques taught to help firefighters come down after traumatic and stressful incidents."

PTSD and suicide

Retired Fire Captain Jeff Dill started the Firefighter Behavioral Health Alliance (FBHA) in 2010, after contacting the U.S. Fire Administration, National Fallen Firefighters Foundation, National Fire Academy, National Volunteer Fire Council, NFPA, National Institute for Occupational Safety and Health, and Occupational Safety and Health Administration, and discovering that none of these agencies kept any data on firefighters and EMS who died by suicide. In 2011, FBHA officially became a 501(c)3 (a not-for-profit entity) and has developed a wide range of workshops and resources specifically for first responders that are targeted toward the stressors they face.

Not only is Dill dedicating his retirement to helping firefighters, he is also up front about how the warrior culture can affect first responders. He explained, "When the public hears the word firefighter, they automatically think of words like brave, strong, courageous, and self-sacrificing. I call this cultural brainwashing because we have these strong psychological associations with professions like firefighting. And while these words certainly apply to firefighters, it's not a balanced perspective." Dill also understands from personal experience how anger can eat away at firefighters:

> I believe anger arises because of all the things firefighters and EMS see and do, over and over. We begin to question society's values, the values of the people we serve. When things don't change or when they get worse, we become negative and start questioning, "How can people treat themselves this way?" "How do they allow themselves to live like this?" You start doubting yourself and what's being asked of you. As a result, you become angry, and this anger infiltrates your family and your relationships. As your relationships deteriorate and your spouse finally walks out the door, you think, "How can you leave me? Everyone loves firefighters! Why would you want to walk away?" And that anger can turn to depression or murder-suicide. Since 2002, we've had 59 validated reports of fire and EMS that have killed their loved one and then killed themselves.

What does Dill think about yoga? He told me he's a firm believer that first responders have to practice self-care, which is "different for so many people—could be journaling, painting, exercise. I really like yoga because while I'm stretching, breathing, and holding

When you put on the uniform, you're expected by the public and your family to always behave in a certain way. Twenty-four hours a day, 7 days a week, firefighters are held to the highest expectations by their fellow brothers and sisters, the community they serve, and the traditions of the fire and EMS culture. But when you are struggling with calls or personal issues, it's very difficult to also be held to these expectations.

—Jeff Dill, retired captain,
Palatine Rural Fire Protection District, Inverness, IL

a position, I can ask myself, 'What's going on right now with my mind and my body?' Yoga helps not just physically, but also with the mind."

Trait 2: Using Systems Thinking

Systems thinking refers to a broad understanding of the intricate coordination of how the mind and body work together (see also chapter 12). At the organizational level, it's the opposite of thinking you have to do it all alone, that it all falls on your shoulders. This is one of the most widely used approaches to enhancing how organizations and systems of any kind function. Systems thinking encourages us to see outside the box to find new ways of solving problems and then manage change more successfully throughout an organization. I've been so impressed with the leaders I've talked to who know how to navigate all the moving parts, from the local to the state level, while reaching out to find innovative ways to respond to crises and serve the mission of the fire service.

A hierarchy really functions as a whole

Matt Samson, deputy chief of the South San Francisco Fire Department, worked with a Red Cross ambulance crew in Spain when he was first out of college. In our interview, he talked about how working somewhere else—with a different language, different system, even a different body language—influenced his development as a leader. "Seeing how people do something with the same end goal, but very differently, allows the brain to see new perspectives," he told me. "There's not just one way."

Samson has taken that open mindset and combined it with an in-depth look at how individual firefighters can have a positive impact at every level. "As a captain, you spend your first year nervous about whether someone will get hurt because you made a bad decision," Samson explained. "Then you start thinking about ways to improve your crews, your own performance. As you get comfortable at this level, you start to see how you can impact the whole department. Then as a battalion chief, you're responsible for the department and the city. That means empowering each captain in the district to be confident thinkers, not just reactors to situations. Now that I'm deputy chief, I'm focusing almost entirely at the global level, budgeting and allocating resources to support our overall mission."

At his level of responsibility, Samson is looking even more widely at how the fire service is affected by changing economic trends. Because his department is in one of the most expensive cities in the United States, Samson is sensitive to the skyrocketing costs of living for the firefighters in his department. "Thirty years ago, every firefighter had a South San Francisco address," Samson said, "and if they didn't, people wondered why not. Today the cost of living is so high that firefighters can't afford to live in the communities they serve. When you lose the community connection, you can lose the way that the fire department gained its reputation. However, our folks do an incredible job of making the effort to connect with the community every chance they get."

Seeing patterns

Leaders skilled in systems thinking are really good at seeing patterns, similarities, crossover possibilities, and how something in one system can be used in another. Examples include borrowing from one system to solve problems in your own, or seeing patterns of failure and not being afraid to acknowledge them and try something different.

As a union president, Dave Gillotte is used to juggling all the systems affecting the California fire service. Of course, keeping these working together has become more fraught during the coronavirus pandemic. When social distancing meant that the Los Angeles County Fire Department was looking at canceling their training program for new recruits, just when they were most needed to fight COVID-19, Gillotte and his team did a quick pivot. Working together, labor and management designed a new program that shortened the training period from 16 to 8 weeks, while maintaining the necessary training and incorporating the distancing and safety guidelines.

Gillotte's department reached out to the military to get ideas. First, drill-tower training would be continued, incorporating new protocols. (Drill towers are concrete and metal structures that give firefighters experience in real-life situations like ladder drills, pump drills, hose management, rope rescue, and working safely at heights and close quarters.) Instructors and trainees are now sequestered, as in the military, but in hotels near the training center.

Rather than one large group, there are smaller groups in different locations to allow proper distance to be maintained. For up-close work, everyone uses N95 respirator masks. As part of the training routine, when the bell signaling to begin the cleaning routine is rung, every piece of equipment is sanitized. Some of this training is conducted online, which cuts down on group interactions. Then, the last two weeks of the program are done at the station where the recruits will be working rather than at the training facility. This means more responsibility falls to the station captains, but as Gillotte explained, Los Angeles County firefighters are adapting.

Before COVID-19, Gillotte was leading the way in bringing yoga into the training program: "We're fighting the battle to get yoga into the drill tower," he told me. "This is the future, and we're damaging our people less if we work them out correctly and focus on job-specific tasks: Can they pull ceilings, pull hose, lift heavy weights in the way we need them to? There are movements in yoga that absolutely mirror our job performance."

Gillotte has done his homework on the benefits of yoga for tactical athletes: "We will continue to ensure that the cardiac output and respiratory capacity and range of motion that come from yoga and similar training practices are part of our program, similar to what major professional sports programs are doing. We must adapt and improve how we do things."

Trait 3: Creating Trust

With first responders, the bullshit detector is very finely tuned—when you're risking your life every day, you like to know who has your back. Terms like "EAP," or "innovation," or "mandatory training" can provoke an instantaneous knee-jerk reaction opposite to their intended direction. I know this because I've been subjected to some pretty intense scrutiny over years as I've grown my business. FireFlex Yoga has earned its outstanding reputation because the first principle I teach in the training program is respect for the fire culture and firefighters. All the leaders I've written about in this chapter understand that without earning the trust of their firefighters, no change initiative will be successful.

Keeping programs relevant and tactical

Deputy Fire Chief Eric Vollmer has been careful to create programs that earn the trust of firefighters. This caution stems from a prior negative experience when his own captain was killed during a training accident at a midsize fire department in the San Francisco Bay Area. "You can't have someone on a peer support team or use a counselor who doesn't have respect within the department because no one will listen honestly and participate openly," he said.

Vollmer's department's peer support program is made up of well-respected firefighters from a wide background. As he described, "Some members are newer and come from the military, and they've experienced this new conversation and seen the value. Some members are firefighters with 20-plus years on a busy ride, meaning they experience their share of bad calls. One member of the team is very religious and approaches the issues from the spiritual side, and others aren't religious at all."

For years, Vollmer has been advocating for the fire service to offer a combination of yoga and mindfulness in firehouses. As he explained, "When your head's not right and you're reacting to an abnormal event or tough day at work, a practice like yoga is going to reduce the release of stress hormones. Deep breathing exercises are going to reduce your blood pressure and heart rate and start the recovery process."

When asked to describe how these practices help on a difficult call, Vollmer said, "I've trained myself to recognize what's going on in my body, so if I pull up to the scene and it's bad and my immediate reaction is, oh crap, or I feel myself getting angry, I take a couple of deep breaths and reset. Just making a commitment to changing my mindset helps, and immediately I see the situation from a new set of eyes. The practices allow you to focus without being overwhelmed."

> To actually get firefighters to come in for some help, they need to feel they can talk to someone who can truly relate and listen without being judgmental.
>
> —Eric Vollmer, deputy fire chief,
> special operations,
> Hayward, CA, Fire Department

Being authentic means walking the talk

David Dolson, division chief and head of training for the Roseville Fire Department in California, has 27 years as a firefighter, most in the city of Sacramento, one of the busiest departments in the country. Dolson is also a certified yoga instructor who's been teaching for eight years. At a very athletic six feet tall, he rarely receives any pushback about yoga not fitting into the fire culture when he teach a class at a fire station.

Dolson teaches one of the modules in my teacher training program. He's a great communicator because he comes from a place of deep personal commitment to walking the talk. He started doing yoga 11 years ago to heal knee and ankle injuries that were affecting him on the job, but he continued because it helped him change his life and perspective.

Years ago, Dolson was struggling with challenges resulting from the intense physical, mental, and emotional demands of working in a busy department and system. Friends and family noticed that he was becoming uptight. "Practicing yoga made me admit I needed help," Dolson reflected. "It helped me see how [being] negative and/or avoiding coping was just allowing things to build up."

Now that he is in a leadership position, Dolson uses yoga and mindfulness practices not only to continue his personal growth but also to keep communication open with his team:

> Yoga practice helps us grow our own personal awareness and then our professional awareness, with each other, with our co-workers, with everyone we interact with. Like our dispatchers, who want to know the outcome of critical calls. It really weighs on them not knowing if a child is still alive, for example. Whatever level someone is operating on, the task level or command level, on the yoga mat we're all the same.

In one of our conversations, Dolson said something that eloquently brought together the values of yoga and the fire culture: "As you grow your experience and wisdom and intelligence, you start understanding that your gut feeling, that intuition that comes from working as a team, is what's going to save your life and keep you safe."

Trait 4: Leading by Example— Self-Regulation and Self-Awareness

In "Command Presence: What Is It, and How Do You Develop It?" Thomas Warren describes leaders with presence and self-awareness: "When they arrive at the scene of a fire or other emergency, everyone knows that they will bring order to the chaos of the emergency scene, and everyone will be safe. In short, they have a kind of authority that is easily recognized and respected by everyone on scene—civilians and firefighters alike."[4] Leaders with a strong sense of self-awareness know themselves, are able to evaluate themselves and the decisions they make objectively—exercising the reflection piece of the readiness framework that Jason Brezler talked about in the introduction to this book, regulating emotions, aligning behavior with values, and recognizing the impact they have on others. It's not a "take it or leave it" attitude. Self-awareness is one of the key traits of emotional intelligence. It's also one of the key benefits you get from practicing interoceptive yoga.

Leading yourself first

All the leaders I've worked with understand that the only person you can really lead is yourself. They've faced their own challenges on the job and aren't afraid to talk about them. They're committed to making physical and mental resilience programs easily available to every firefighter and, most importantly, making it acceptable to ask for help. By doing that, they lead by example.

In chapter 1, I told Battalion Chief Jason Golden's inspiring story about how he and his colleagues pioneered a program to help firefighters and the community after the devastating wildfires in California in 2017. Golden's passionate advocacy for both physical and mental fitness had its beginnings when he was a young firefighter and had to perform

CPR on his deputy chief in the station. Golden said it was a number of years before he was able to admit to himself how badly he was affected, not just by the death of his chief but also by the ongoing stress of the job. He finally sought help, which opened his eyes to the wider need for this kind of support within the fire culture. There was a moment, Golden told me, when he thought to himself, "Hey, I can either hide my secret of needing help, or I can be candid about my own pain, and thereby let my agency know there's an urgent need for mental health support for firefighters." Golden stepped up and chose the latter path. Even though he was afraid of being ostracized or looked at differently, he recalls that the exact opposite happened: "A lot of people have come forward to say they're suffering and wondering how they can get help."

In addition to therapy, Golden credits yoga and mindfulness practices for helping him be a better leader:

> Yoga really helped me to quiet everything down because when we're at work we're constantly on the go and at a heightened state of awareness. It's important to take that time to slow things down and take a breather. Learning the breathing exercises was really important because when the tones go off, I'll literally take a deep breath and feel my body calm down. I can think more clearly when I have to make decisions that are going to affect my crew, that are going to affect the public.

Self-care is a strength

Fire Chief Sam DiGiovanna of the Verdugo Fire Academy in Los Angeles has been practicing yoga and mindfulness for more than 15 years, starting back when yoga was definitely not part of the warrior culture and doing stretches on a yoga mat or meditating were considered weird. He credits these techniques with supporting leadership skills like mental and physical flexibility, being able to let go of negative thoughts, and having better concentration, composure, and decision-making during high-stress events, whether fires, labor issues, or combative city council meetings.

DiGiovanna reflected on a pivotal leadership experience he had shortly after being appointed interim fire chief. This highlighted for him the importance of self-care techniques like yoga:

> There was a Santa Ana wind blowing at approximately 40 mph with 60 mph gusts. We had multiple calls of wires down, trees uprooted, power outages, et cetera. Then the tones went off for a brush fire in the west side of town, immediately followed by tones for a brush fire in the east end. Two working brush fires in the same town, with units starting to report smoke quite a ways out from the west-side fire, and the engine working the east side reporting multiple fires on the roofs of surrounding houses. Thinking "I'm about to lose half my community," I remembered "Breathe! Don't stress, no monkey chatter—just a clear mind, unattached." With a clearer head I quickly started ordering additional strike teams and began strategically assigning resources. Certainly through the grace of God and surrounded with highly skilled personnel, the fires were put out.

As a champion of yoga, DiGiovanna is pleased that so many more firefighters are experiencing the benefits. "Yoga seemed complicated at first, but it really isn't," he told me. "It's really about unlearning old ways and habits of dealing with stress and difficult situations and replacing them with simple, mindful techniques and breathing exercises."

Leading as One of the 4%

Each of the women I've written about in this chapter is a total badass, and so is my sister Deputy Fire Marshall Tracey Oliver. I admire them not only because they thrive in one of the most dangerous and male-dominated professions in the country, one where strength is not just a necessity but a virtue, but also because of their fearlessness in mixing it up with what are considered feminine attributes—compassion, collaboration, communication, and my favorite, using your mind to leverage your power. What do I mean by this? Here are some stories from the women I've interviewed and worked with who are part of the 4%.

Work smarter not stronger

Let's start with hose management. When Oliver was still a probationary firefighter, her captain decided to make her the hose management *train the trainer*—learning the skill through teaching it to recruits at the academy. "Charged fire hoses have a lot of pressure or force," Oliver told me. "Most guys try to use brute strength to deal with it. My captain showed me some technical procedures for managing the force generated by the water flow to save energy and make the job easier. Then when I showed new recruits how to do it and how you can even put the hose bend against the wall to take away some of the force, they looked at me like, 'Wow! Work smarter not stronger!'"

Teamwork: not everyone has to carry the axe

As a fire engineer at Healdsburg Fire Department in Sonoma County (CA), Amanda Newhall is responsible for all of their vehicles: four-wheel-drive wildland trucks, a water tender (which resembles a portable fire hydrant), a ladder truck, and two type 1 fire engines. The department answers calls for the municipal airport, provides mutual aid to the Sonoma County Airport, and responds to swiftwater river rescues, wildland and structure fires, freeway extrications, and vehicle accidents—and don't forget the 2017 and 2019 wildfires! Her department also shares fire duties with other departments, so Newhall has honed her skills in collaboration and teamwork, particularly when she's part of an out-of-county fire deployment.

Newhall told me that with regular assignments, she has a great team where they've established who should be doing what based on specific strengths and what works best. As she put it, "Who should be carrying the axe and who should be carrying the Halligan hook."

Strike teams—out-of-county deployments including several engines of the same type and one leader—are tougher, observed Newhall. "I stick out a bit more because I'm usually the only female on the fire line, which often includes spending the night in a base camp. As part of Sonoma County, we might have five different departments [responding together], so getting them to trust me and me to trust them is the challenge."

When I asked Newhall how she manages this, her answer cracked me up: "There's always going to be some butt-sniffing as soon as someone who doesn't belong walks in," she said. I totally got what she was saying because back in 2014, I experienced the same behavior when

> Yoga is the most efficient tool we have to address the NFPA health and wellness standards.
>
> —Amanda Newhall, fire engineer
> at Healdsburg, CA,
> Fire Department

I entered a new firehouse to start a yoga program—but doing it in a wilderness base camp with a devastating wildfire all around you? Newhall went on to explain, "I've never had a problem we couldn't figure out, not to the point when I wasn't able to handle it. It's a matter of clear communication and establishing where everyone is so we can do our job well and feel safe around each other." It doesn't get more badass than that!

Yoga in the mix

As her department's safety officer, which includes responsibility for health and wellness, Newhall is a big advocate of yoga for supporting resiliency, particularly when "things get dark and you need the tools to navigate this [darkness]." One reason Newhall likes yoga and mindfulness so much is because you can take the practices on the road:

> I do a lot of yoga stretches, even five minutes of sun salutations, on the fire line or at base camp. Making time for my body and my mental state is especially important when I'm on campaign incidents or out on long deployments where you're stuck in a tiny type 3 engine with a few other people and after three weeks you're really getting on each other's nerves. When you take a few minutes to do yoga, things shift and you get grounded, and remember who you are—not just a tired, hungry person.

Tracey Oliver is also a proponent of yoga. She has a degree in kinesiology, she's a certified strength and conditioning specialist with the National Strength and Conditioning Association, and she's a certified personal trainer. Naturally, I asked her to review this writing and to get her take on how yoga benefits firefighters. She started practicing yoga to heal a non–work-related back injury. As long as she did her exercises, there was no more back pain, she said.

Jenn Panko likes the holistic approach that yoga brings to an overall wellness program. In her words, "The more fit you are mentally and physically, the safer you'll be, the fewer injuries you'll have, the longer your career will be, and the more stress relief you'll have."

In sum, how do I think women are leading in the fire service? I see them as bringing a new authenticity to the profession. They are unafraid to be themselves. They balance both masculine and feminine attributes in a way that's not threatening but definitely shows that they can handle the "heat" at any level. In fact, some of the firefighters in Panko's department coined the phrase, "to get Panko'd," to describe any situation where her tenacity in getting the attention of leadership resulted in projects getting done. I took this as a sign of respect for her ability to make things happen.

Through their competency in the field and their commitment to the profession, female firefighters demonstrate that a diversity of skills and talents adds power and better problem solving at any level of the fire service. With the demands of the new fire service calling for cooperation and communication more than competition—that is, where survival of the fittest isn't the rule anymore—women are leading the way forward.

Trait 5: Compassion—the Key to Leading

Acknowledge your inner critic, then tell it to shut the hell up

I was recently on a hike with my husband, Tom, in the mountains surrounding Lake Tahoe. The first three miles of the hike were uphill. I was tired, but my first response was to let my inner critic kick in: "So what if you're tired! Suck it up!" I gritted my teeth and started climbing, setting a pace that was more punishing than enjoyable. When I finally recognized what was happening, I gave myself permission to remember the words of "Martin," the wise and highly experienced trail guide for a six-day trek I did in Yosemite: "Pace yourself" was his mantra.

Martin was a big man, over six feet tall, and he had mapped out a number of backcountry trails in Yosemite. Martin never walked faster than a stroll. When I finally asked the rationale behind his saunter, he explained that this strategy allowed him to work smart: stay in the present moment, conserve his strength, be situationally aware at all times. This is how he was able to lead treks up to dangerous peaks like El Capitan all summer long, successfully logging hundreds of miles every summer. This is how he could add additional duties during these arduous trips, like cooking breakfast, lunch, and dinner and then cleaning up; smoothing out family squabbles; lightening the mood by telling jokes to keep the "brand-new-boots" city folk who wanted to become weekend warriors from flagging.

Remembering this influence, I decided to pace myself at Lake Tahoe. Once I slowed down, I didn't have to spend all my attention analyzing the trail, worrying about tripping and twisting an ankle or whether I had the energy to make it to the top. Instead, I had time to observe my other thoughts, the ones I was keeping at bay by powering through my hike. And I didn't like what I found: a swirling stream of judgments and critiques in which I berated myself for not being more successful; rehearsed a victorious conversation where I cut my friend to the quick; imagined my father's funeral, which at the time I knew was imminent, and wondering what I would wear. Nice, Shannon!

What to do with this relentless inner critic? I focused on being more attentive to what was happening in the moment: my feet hitting the soft dirt, the pine needles crunching under my boots, the chirping of squirrels and birds—sensations that a few moments before had been obscured by my inner dialogue.

The most amazing result of focusing on what's happening in the moment rather than on your negative thoughts is that it allows other feelings to come to the forefront—for example, curiosity, humor, and joy. Suddenly I had more energy, and now in a playful mood, I quickly overtook my husband on the trail, glancing back at him with a sly smile. I didn't say my competitive nature completely disappeared!

The lesson we learn over and over from practicing yoga and mindfulness is that you can get a handle on the nonstop monologue of the inner critic. Once you isolate that inner voice, you can choose to listen or tell it to shut the hell up! Because the truth is, we are not our thoughts. We actually have dominion over them. This is the beginning of leading from a place of compassion, strength, and resilience.

How is this compassion?

When the Dalai Lama met with teachers of mindfulness in the West in 1989, they were discussing metta, a meditation practice roughly translated as loving kindness that embraces the feeling of benevolence or compassion for all others to be happy, healthy, and free from suffering (see chapter 12).

In metta practice in the West, you start by sending feelings of compassion to yourself, which in English is known as *self-compassion*. The Dalai Lama was curious about the inclusion of the word "self" in this term, because in the East, the practice of compassion automatically includes oneself. It was explained that because self-loathing is so pervasive in the West, people had to be reminded that they, like everyone else, are worthy and deserving of compassion and kindness.[5]

For first responders, who are expected to live up to the warrior code, self-compassion is even tougher. All the firefighters I describe in this chapter are leaders who are just ordinary people trying in their own ways to make things better. One of the reasons I admire them so much is that they share this trait of compassion for themselves as well as for others.

Former Police Lieutenant Richard Goerling, a pioneer of mindfulness for first responders, explains how training compassion, both internally and externally, is synonymous with surviving your shift. They are, in fact, synchronized.

Goerling used to believe that demonstrating compassion for others would make him less of a badass warrior and could jeopardize his safety, potentially his life. However, once he began to learn more about mindfulness, including the key components of self-study and compassion, he realized that these are foundational skills in all areas of a first responder's life. You can be an officer who can enforce the law, maintain the peace, and care for the safety and well-being of others while at the same attending to your own personal safety and well-being.[6]

In fact, research is showing that metta can reduce depression and PTSD symptoms among veterans.[7] In addition, it quiets the inner critic and increases emotional intelligence.[8] One study found that just seven minutes of practice boosts a person's positive feelings and sense of social connection.[9] Importantly, having social connections is considered a key element of resiliency.

Goerling points out, though, that most first responder departments aren't clamoring to sign up for these kinds of programs. The old warrior culture still has a hold, and compassion often remains seen as a weakness or liability. However, things are changing, and it starts with "self-leadership."

Leading by example

It turns out, the only person you can actually lead is yourself. Then, people need to have the free will, the choice, to follow. Coercing, duping, or forcing people is not leadership, and following by choice is showing respect.

For example, throughout my life my father smoked cigarettes. He knew it was a nasty habit and addictive, and he didn't want any of us kids to start smoking. However, it's a behavior we saw my dad engage in all day long. We loved him and looked up to him. He implored us not to smoke, often with a cigarette in his mouth! He even offered us money if we promised not to start smoking before we turned 18. Three out of four started smoking before this age, so not only did we not get the money, but we also had to figure out how to quit.

"Do what I say, not what I do" is something I hear all the time in the fire departments. I typically start my pitch for yoga in the fire station by presenting department chiefs with the research, results, and positive feedback from firefighter participants; this makes a powerful case, and most fire chiefs give us the green light. However, once the program starts, we rarely see the chief.

Fire chiefs don't join classes because they're too busy. But everyone is aware of who is in class and who opted out. When that person is the head of the organization, what message does it send to the troops? Essentially, yoga—and therefore self-care—is not a priority or an essential part of leadership.

Let's contrast this leadership style with Chief Ruben Torres, who once worked with my dad in San Jose and now leads the Santa Clara Fire Department. We started, as we do at 90% of our departments, with a 10-session program. Chief Torres participated in eight of these sessions, which meant driving to the training center to attend. Consequently, this department has one of our most successful programs, with more than 50% of participants improving their FMS score and 100% requesting additional FireFlex Yoga programs.

The conscious warrior

So many of the stories of leadership in this chapter are about firefighters taking the chance to be vulnerable—to talk about their anxiety, their fear, and their shadow side—or simply taking the chance to do something differently. Would they be ostracized? Looked at differently? Thought of as weak? Passed over for promotion? They did it anyway and changed themselves and their departments, in ways both big and small. They are examples of the conscious warrior I see emerging everywhere in the fire service.

Everyone I interviewed and worked with talked about yoga, mindfulness, and breathing exercises as tools to cut through the clutter, manage anxiety, and focus their attention. In honesty, we're all afraid, and first responders have to deal with not only their personal hang-ups, but society's as well. By seeking out the interventions they need for themselves, these conscious warriors signal the crucial understanding that getting depressed, having anxiety, and suffering a traumatic injury are all normal repercussions of the job and of being human.

Most important, through their actions, these conscious warriors signal that firefighters don't want pity, they don't need to be rescued, and they absolutely don't want to be thought of as broken when they get injured, physically or psychologically. What they do want is access to training that normalizes the consequences of being in a public safety career for 20–30 years. They want tools that lead to the outcomes laid out in this book: better resilience, an open mindset, more self-awareness and compassion, less stress, and better well-being—at work and in their personal lives.

My Thanks and Gratitude!

It's been my privilege and the best part of my career to have made the connection between the work of first responders and the need for yoga and mindfulness training. After going down this road for more than seven years, not knowing whether yoga would be just another fad in the fire service or change the way firefighters and other first responders train for all areas of their lives, I can proudly say that we are moving slowly but steadily toward full integration, using yoga as part of the solution for the crisis in the fire service.

What might full integration look like? Based on the exciting progress being made, especially in the past few years, I see programs like FireFlex Yoga reaching departments throughout the country. I see yoga becoming an integral part in support of every behavioral health and wellness program. I see healthier, high-performing firefighters who are conscious warriors, able to lead with grace under fire. By living this way, they will be able to pay it forward.

14

The Yoga Challenge

Welcome to the yoga challenge! The challenge is known as WOW, for Workout of the Week. This is similar to Workout of the Day, but measured on a weekly basis. Your WOW challenge is to complete five consecutive weeks of yoga poses:

- Week 1: Hip mobility (chapter 8)
- Week 2: Shoulder mobility (chapter 9)
- Week 3: Trunk and joint stability (chapter 10)
- Week 4: The balancing act (chapter 11)
- Week 5: Integration (chapter 12)

Each week has its own sequence, progressing through the goals of the 10-class program outlined in part 5 of this book, and each sequence includes 15–20 poses. However, some of the poses repeat, so it's not as daunting as it might seem. Each sequence is designed to take 30–45 minutes to complete.

This chapter has a section of instructions for each week, introduced by thumbnail pictures of each sequence, as an overview of your progression through the challenge. Keep in mind that I've been doing yoga for more than 20 years, so don't worry if your poses do not look exactly the same!

Each week's sequence builds on the previous one, so jumping around is not advised. Some of the poses that appear to be "easier" are not so simple to do safely. Yoga is about mental as well as physical fitness, so the challenge often comes in your ability to stay present to what you're feeling in your body as you go through the sequences. The challenge is to become your own teacher.

Here's how to start the WOW yoga challenge:

- Pick a starting date
- Review the poses in week 1, then carefully read the instructions for the first pose and begin. Repeat with the next pose.
- Practice the entire sequence three or four times over the week on and off duty. Move to week 2.
- Bonus points if you can inspire your crew or your family to join you!

One more defining trait separating this program from others: most yoga instructors say things like "Hold for five breaths," which is a very prescriptive way to practice. By contrast, FireFlex Yoga is built around interoceptive yoga, which is about choice and empowerment. So these instructions provide a starting point, with the understanding that you can adjust the poses to fit your needs as you get more comfortable with them and attuned to what your body is telling you. So when you are ready, roll out your mat!

Week 1: My Hips Are So Tight!

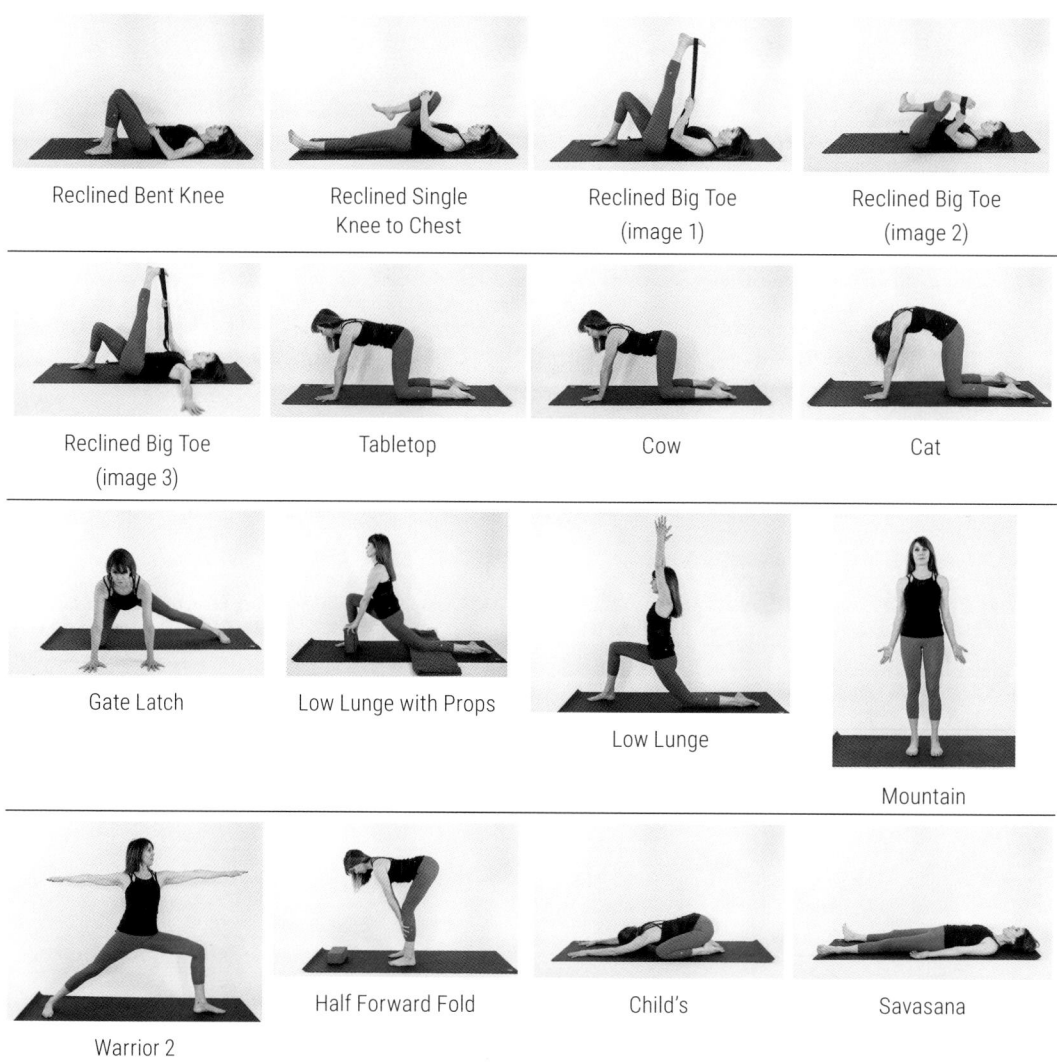

Reclined Bent Knee

Reclined Single Knee to Chest

Reclined Big Toe (image 1)

Reclined Big Toe (image 2)

Reclined Big Toe (image 3)

Tabletop

Cow

Cat

Gate Latch

Low Lunge with Props

Low Lunge

Mountain

Warrior 2

Half Forward Fold

Child's

Savasana

Reclined Bent Knee

1. Start lying on your back. Bend your knees and slide your feet in a comfortable distance from your hips.
2. Hold for a few breaths and note how the pose feels in your body.

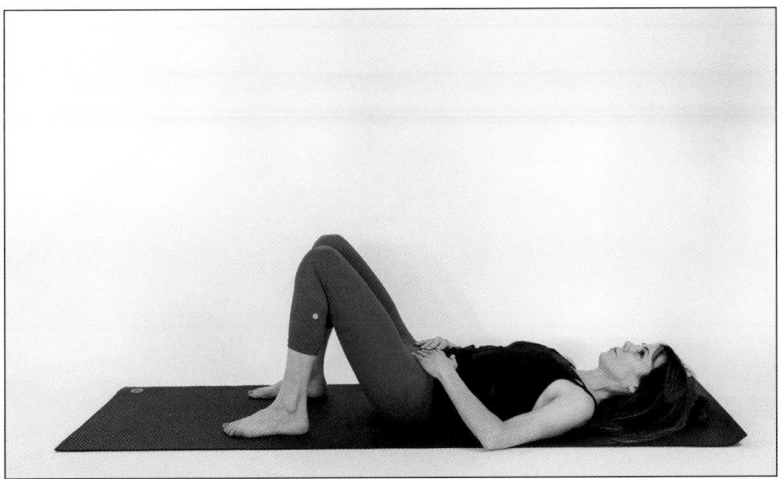

Reclined Single Knee to Chest

1. Start lying on your back with legs extended on the floor. Pull your right knee into your chest and clasp your hands across your shin or behind your knee. Keep your head and upper back in contact with the surface beneath you.
2. Hold for a few breaths and note how the pose feels in your body.
3. Repeat on the opposite side.

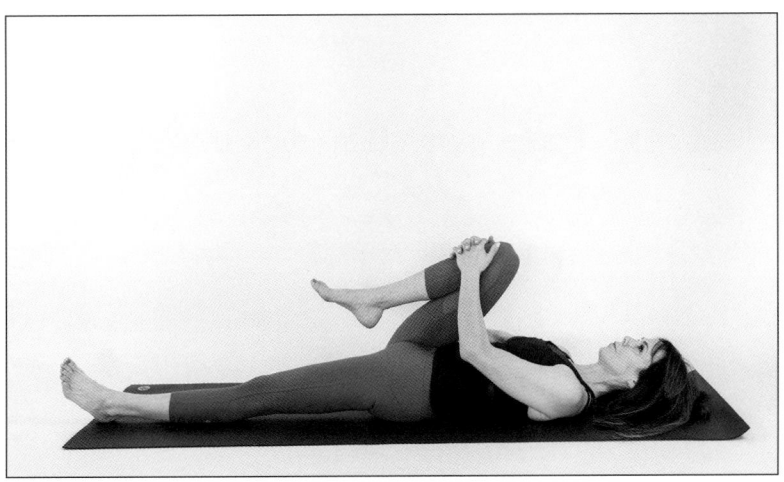

Reclined Big Toe

1. Start lying on your back with knees bent and feet drawn in. Bring your right knee into your chest and wrap a strap around the widest part of your foot.
2. Hold the strap in both hands and begin to straighten your right leg. Move your right hip back to lengthen the right side of the lower back, and square your hips.

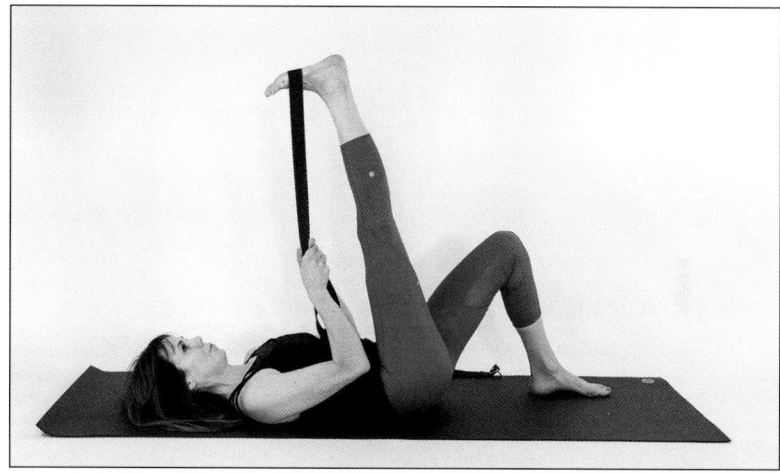

3. Hold for a few breaths and note how the pose feels in your body.
4. Next, hold both ends of the strap in your right hand. Lift your left foot up and draw your left knee toward your right knee. Bring your left hand into the inner left knee and separate your knees by moving your right leg to the right and your left knee to the left. To keep from tipping to one side, distribute your weight evenly across the back of the pelvis.

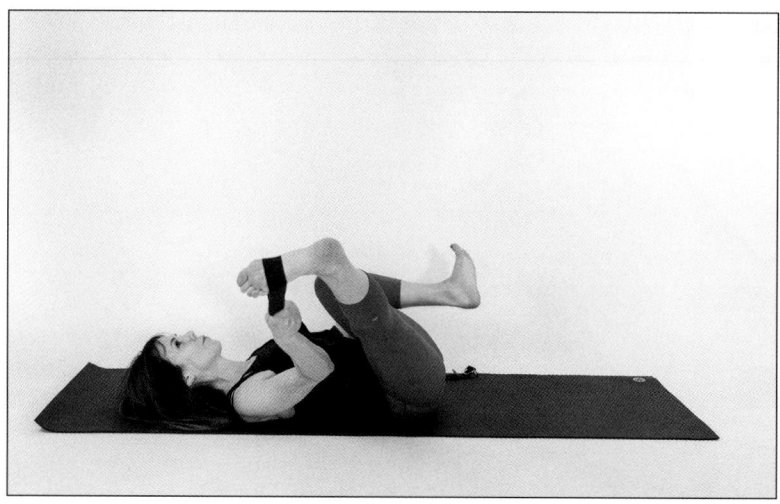

5. Hold for a few breaths and note how the pose feels in your body.

6. Next, draw your knees back together and place your left foot on the mat. Now switch hands with the strap, holding both ends of the strap in the left hand. Place your right thumb in the right hip crease and gently press your hip back as you move the right leg across to the left. Keep the back of your right hip and shoulder in contact with the surface beneath you. Allow your left knee to roll in.

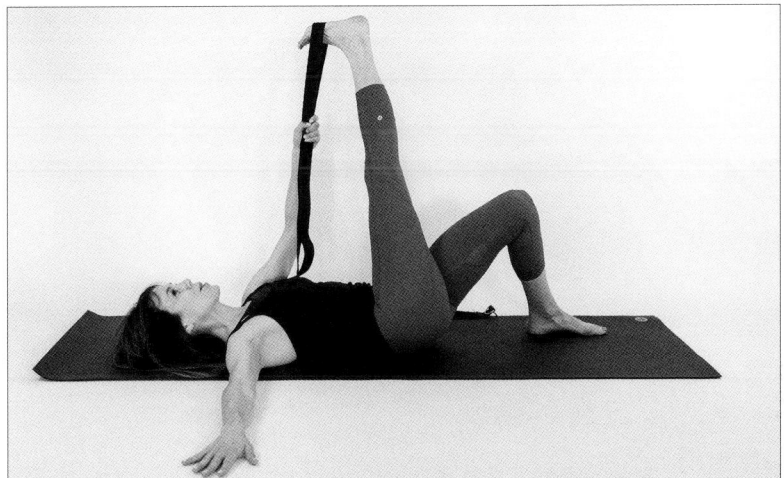

7. Hold for a few breaths and note how the pose feels in your body.
8. Release into reclined bent knee pose and repeat the entire sequence on the opposite side.

Tabletop

1. Start on all fours, with your wrists underneath your shoulders and your knees underneath the hips. Separate your knees hip-width apart, with the feet directly behind the knees. Your knees should stack directly under your hips, with your palms directly under your shoulders. Spread your fingers wide.
2. Hug your belly up and in, so that your lower back doesn't arch. Keep your lower arms in a neutral position and begin to externally rotate and stabilize the shoulder joint by rolling your upper arms away from you. Draw your shoulders firmly against the back of your rib cage, creating more space across your upper back, allowing your neck to relax. Feel your collarbones spread. Gaze down at the floor without dropping your head, keeping the back of your neck long.

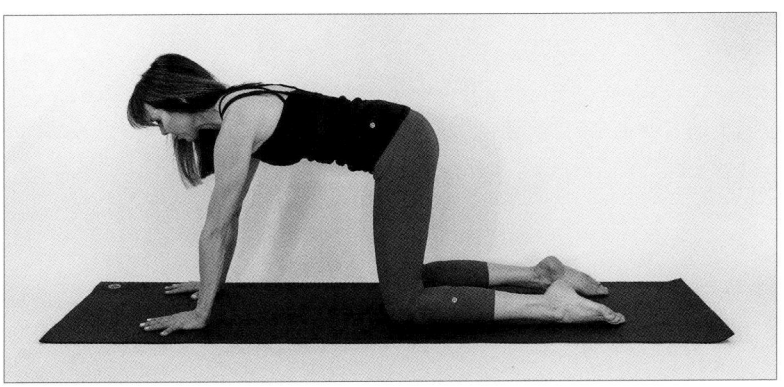

Cow

1. Start in tabletop with wrists under shoulders and knees under hips.
2. Inhale and lift your sitting bones and chest forward and up, then allow your belly to sink toward the floor. Move the front of your shoulders back and feel your shoulder blades move toward your spine. Lift your head to look straight ahead or up toward the ceiling.
3. Exhale, coming back to a neutral tabletop position on your hands and knees.
4. Repeat a few times, noting how the movement feels in your body.

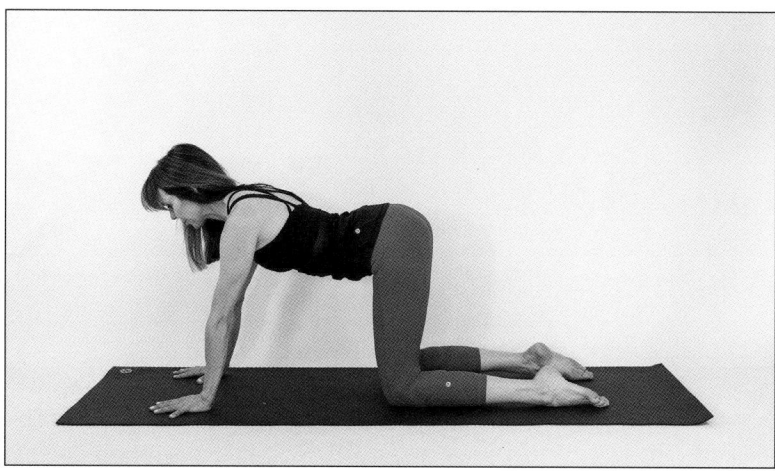

Cat

1. Start in tabletop with wrists under shoulders and knees under hips. Exhale and round your spine toward the ceiling, pulling your belly toward your spine. Release your head toward the floor, but don't force your chin to your chest.
2. Inhale, coming back to a neutral tabletop position on your hands and knees.
3. Repeat a few times, noting how the movement feels in your body.

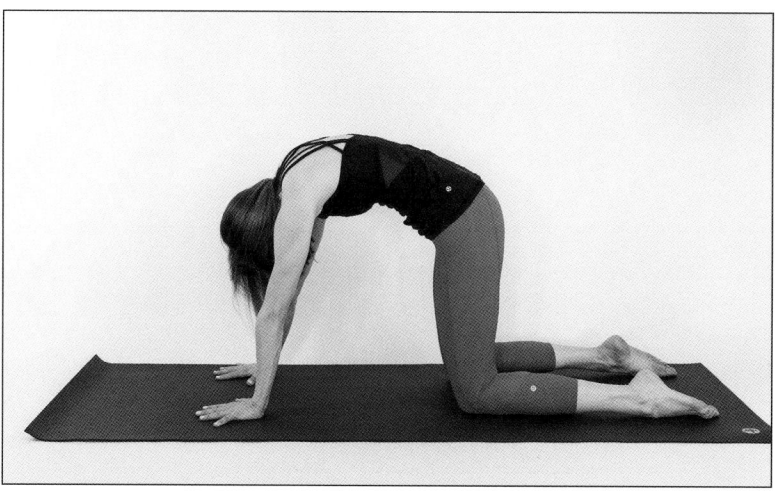

Gate Latch

1. Start in tabletop with wrists under shoulders and knees under hips. Stretch your left leg out to the left. Bring your left ankle and hip in line and press your left foot to the floor, gluing the outer edge of the left foot down. Keep your right knee directly below your right hip (so that your right thigh is perpendicular to the floor).
2. Level your pelvis and hug your belly up and in so that your lower back does not arch.
3. Hold for several breaths and note how the pose feels in your body.
4. Release back into tabletop pose and repeat on the opposite side.

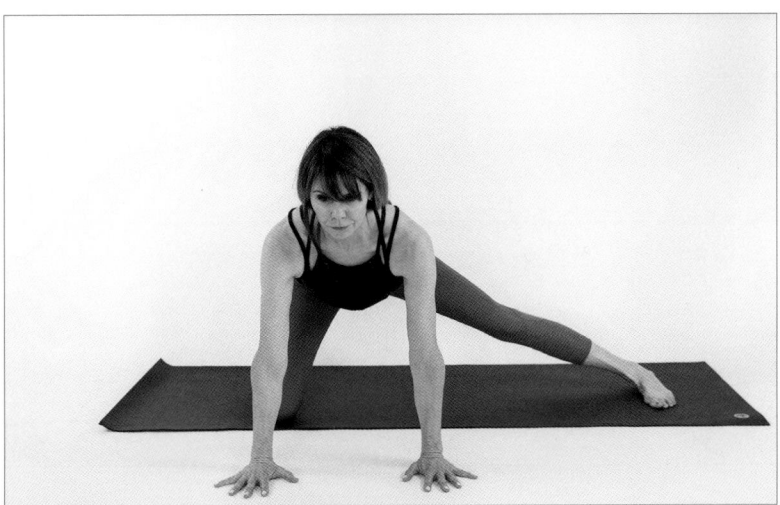

Low Lunge–Low Lunge with Props

1. Start in tabletop with wrists under the shoulders and knees under the hips. Press into your fingertips and tent your palms (or place blocks underneath your hands), and step your right foot forward in between your hands. Stack your right knee over your right heel. If there's too much pressure on the back of your knee, place a blanket or padding underneath the knee and shin.

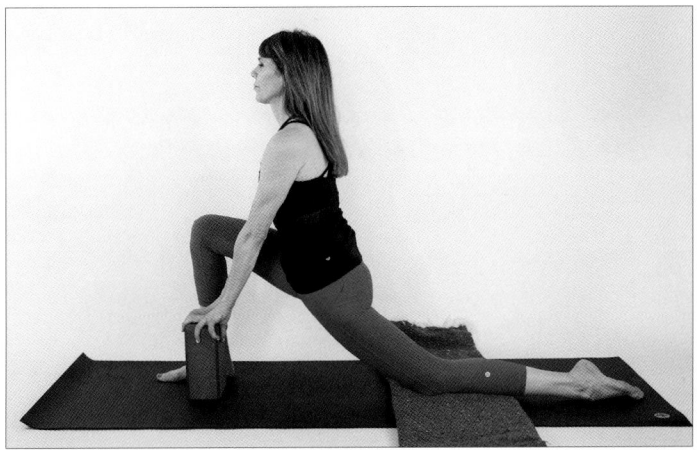

2. Keep your hands down or lift your torso upright to stack shoulders over hips. Your torso and the front of your pelvis are perpendicular to the floor. Angle your tailbone down and place your hands on your hips to level your pelvis.

3. Maintaining a neutral pelvis, release your arms down by your sides. Turn your palms out to externally rotate and stabilize your shoulder joints, then reach your arms out and overhead.

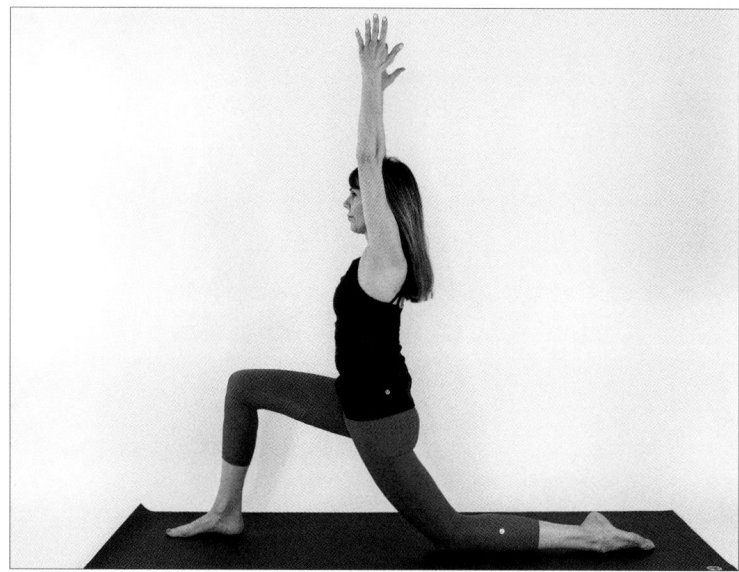

4. Keep your hands shoulder-width apart and allow the tops of your shoulders to release and relax down, away from your ears.

5. Hold for several breaths and note how the pose feels in your body.

6. Release back into tabletop and repeat on the opposite side.

Mountain

1. Start by standing tall, with your feet parallel and hip width apart. Press into the big-toe mound (the pad under the big toe) and pull up through your inner arches.
2. Press your thigh bones back while gently angling your tailbone down. Find a neutral pelvis and a light engagement of the abdomen. Draw your shoulders back to align with your hips and soften the front of the rib cage inward.
3. Stack the crown of your head above your pelvis, with your chin level to the floor. Press down through front, back, inside, and outside of both feet and lift up through the length of your body, feeling the extension through your entire spine.
4. Hold for several breaths and note how the pose feels in your body.

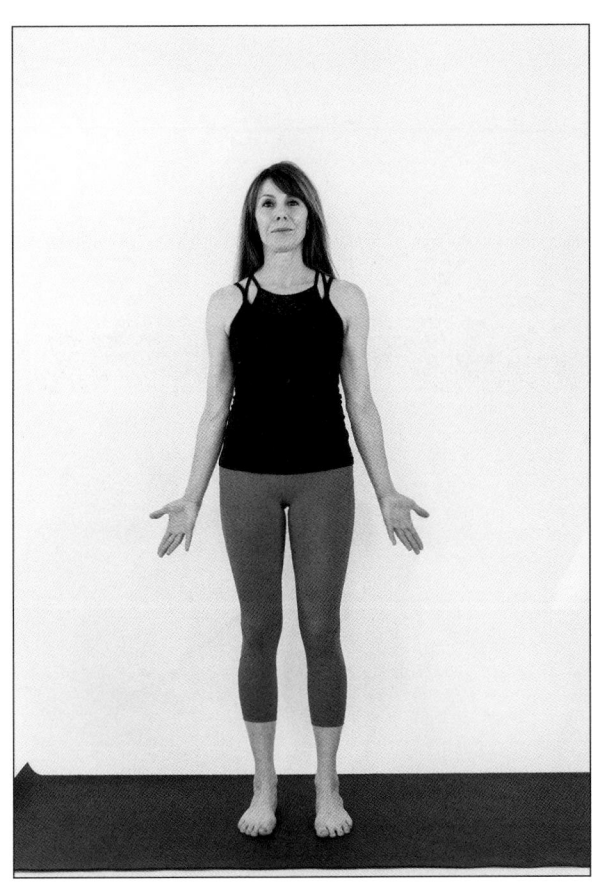

Warrior 2

1. Start by standing tall in mountain. Extend your arms out to the side, shoulder height, like a cross. Separate your feet wide apart, so that your ankles are underneath your wrists.
2. Turn your left toes outward and your right foot slightly inward. Slowly bend your left knee while guiding it toward the little-toe side of the foot, stacking knee above heel. If knee goes beyond heel, increase the distance between your feet.
3. Draw your left sitting bone under. Keep your hips level and pelvis neutral, with your back leg firm. Move your shoulder blades together and down your back, with shoulders stacked above hips.
4. Hold for several breaths and note how the pose feels in your body. Press through your feet to release.
5. Repeat on the opposite side.

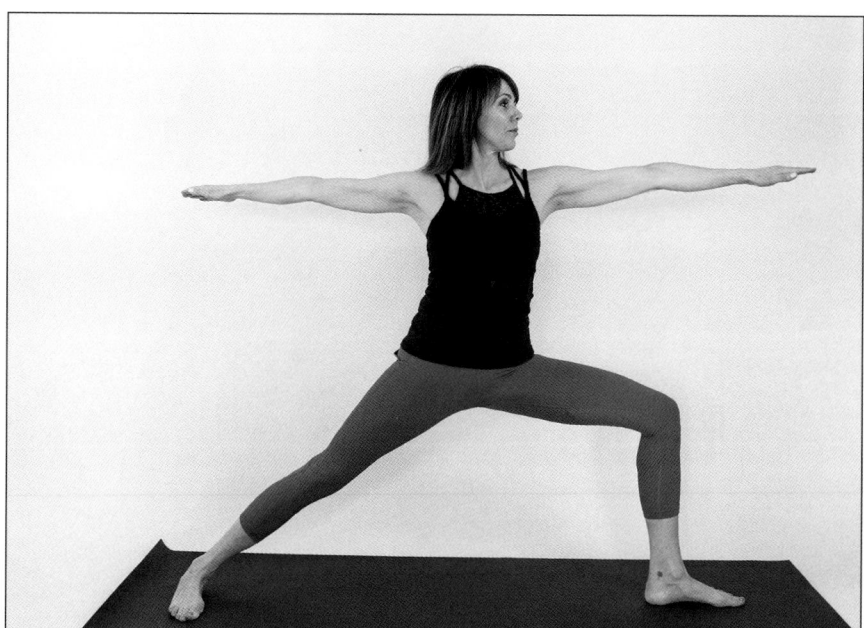

Half Forward Fold

1. Start in Mountain, with your hands on your hips. Soften your knees and feel the weight of your body move into your heels as your hips draw back.
2. Lower your torso forward, making sure the rotation of your pelvis follows your spine. Keep your knees soft and your torso parallel with the floor.
3. Release your hands to your thighs or shins. Lengthen the front of the spine and draw your shoulder blades down your back, keeping your chest lifted and collarbones broad. Focus your gaze on the floor in front of you to release your neck.
4. Hold for several breaths and note how the pose feels in your body.
5. Release by lifting your torso upright and back into mountain.

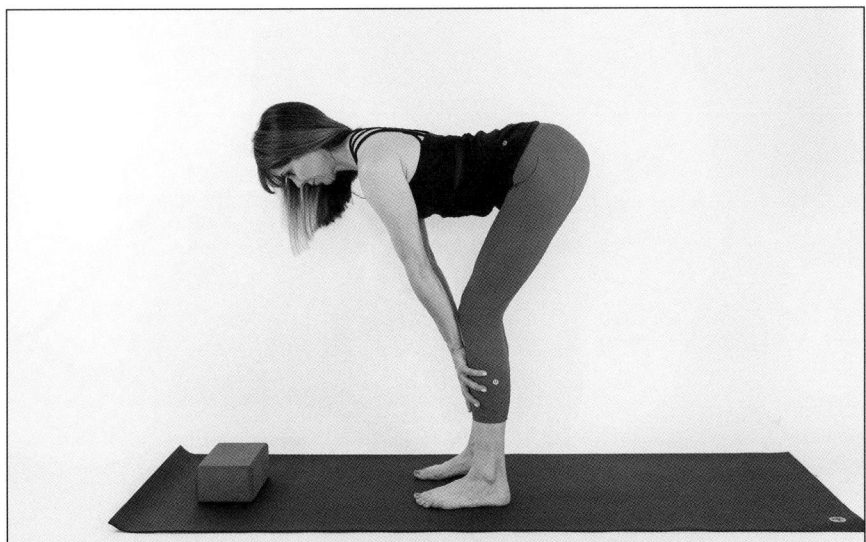

Child's

1. Start in tabletop with wrists under shoulders and knees under hips. Release your hips back toward your heels.
2. Separate your knees wider apart, while keeping your big toes touching to release through the hips, easing pressure in the lower back. Your arms can be draped alongside your legs or out in front of you to reduce pressure in your neck and shoulders.
3. Be mindful of your breathing and note how the pose feels in your body.

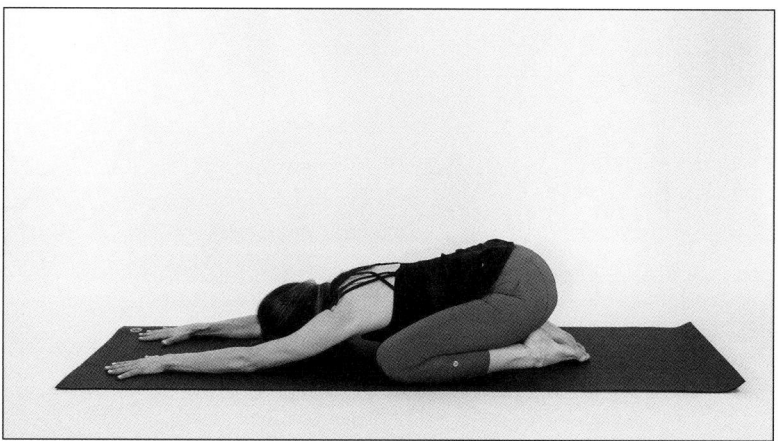

Savasana

1. Start lying on your back, with legs extended. Spread out as comfortably as possible. Drape your arms on the floor, palms facing up. Lift your chest and draw your shoulder blades gently toward your spine. Allow your feet to drop open. Place a rolled-up blanket under your knees to release any discomfort in your back. Take a deep breath and let everything go.
2. Allow your breath to return to its natural rhythm.
3. Stay in this pose for a few minutes after a yoga session or whenever you want to completely relax.

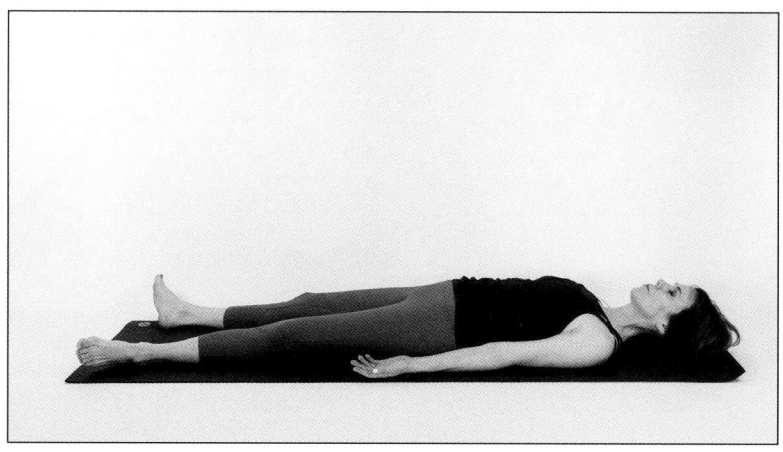

Week 2: Shouldering the Load

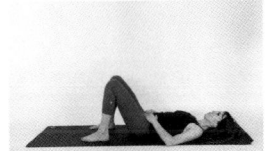

Reclined Bent Knee

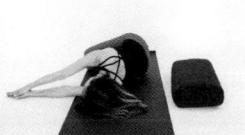

Supine Chest Stretch
(image 1)

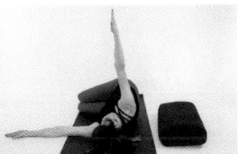

Supine Chest Stretch
(image 2)

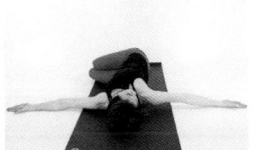

Supine Chest Stretch
(image 3)

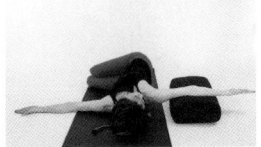

Supine Chest Stretch
(image 4)

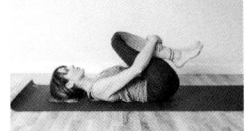

Upward-Facing Child's

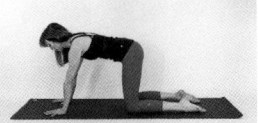

Tabletop

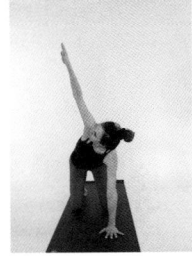

Thread the Needle
(image 1)

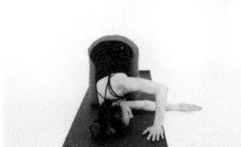

Thread the Needle
(image 2)

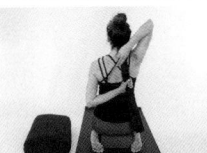

Reciprocal Reaching
Stretch with Strap

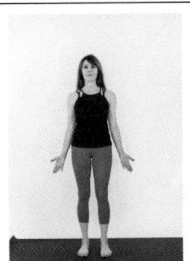

Mountain

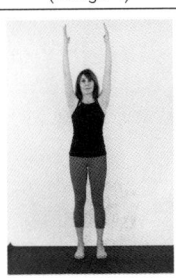

Extended Mountain

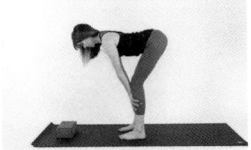

Half Forward Fold

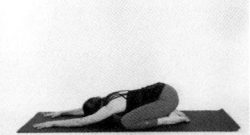

Child's

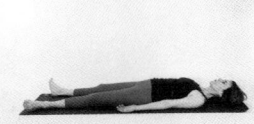

Savasana

Reclined Bent Knee—Supine Chest Stretch

1. Start lying on your back with knees bent.

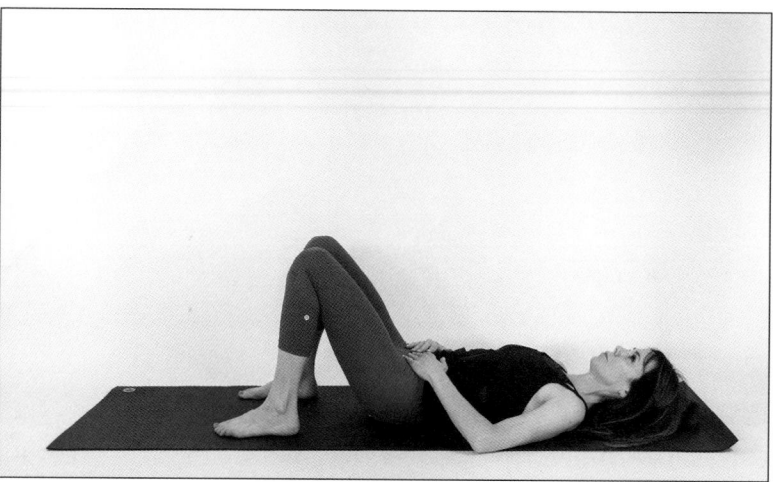

Extend your arms out in the shape of a cross, with your palms facing up. Roll onto your left side in a fetal position and stack your palms. Rest your head on your left ear.

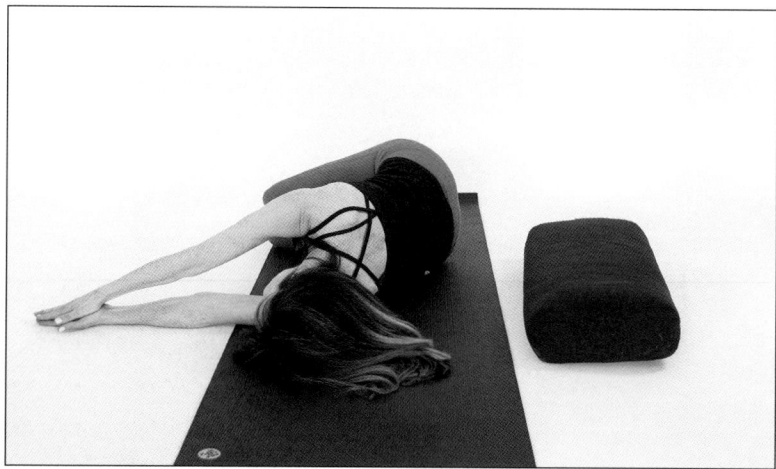

2. Without moving your lower body, inhale and lift your right arm up, fingertips pointing to the ceiling and arms forming a 90° angle. Let your head move along with your arm.

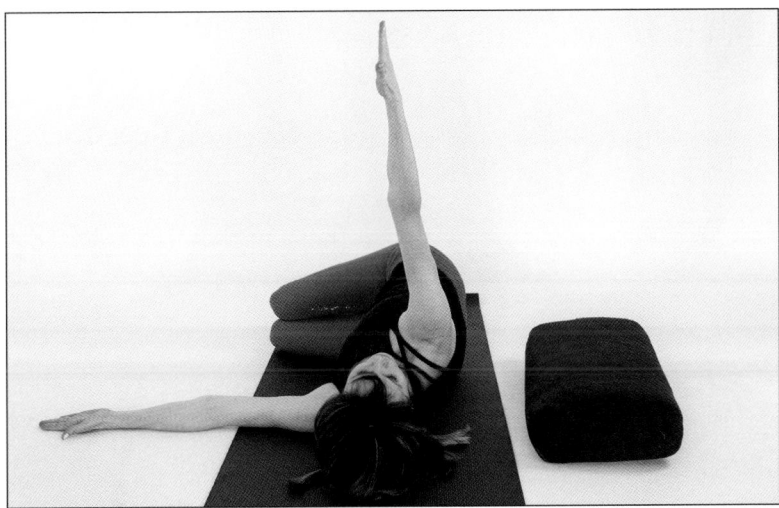

3. Exhaling, continue moving your right arm in an arc behind you, your head following, until your right shoulder and shoulder blade are in contact with the floor (or as close as you can comfortably get). Stretch across your chest and right shoulder.

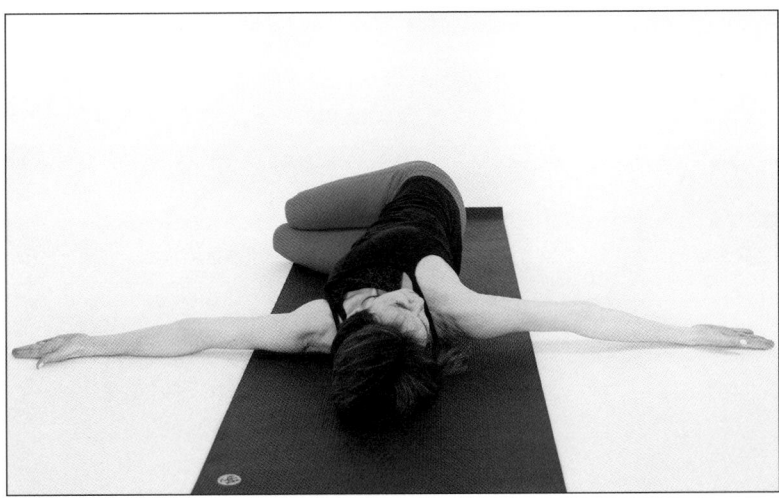

4. If your right arm and hand are suspended, consider placing a firm bolster or block under your right arm, easing tension in your upper back and neck.

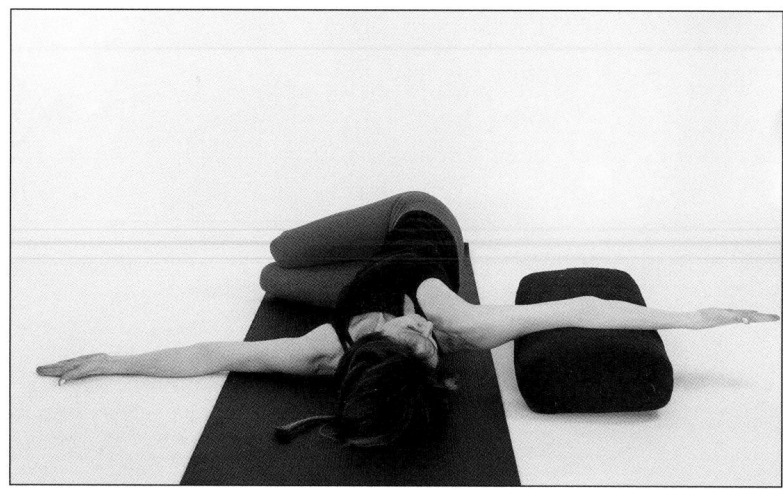

5.   Release back into the starting position. Repeat a few times, moving with your breath, and noting how the pose feels in your body.

6.   Repeat the entire sequence on the other side.

Upward-Facing Child's

1.   Start lying on your back. Bend your knees and slide your feet in at a comfortable distance from your hips. Draw your knees into your chest, one at a time.

2.   Clasp your hands behind your knees or across your shins, keeping your upper back and the back of your head in contact with the floor. Experiment by rocking side to side or moving your knees in a circle to release tension from your lower back.

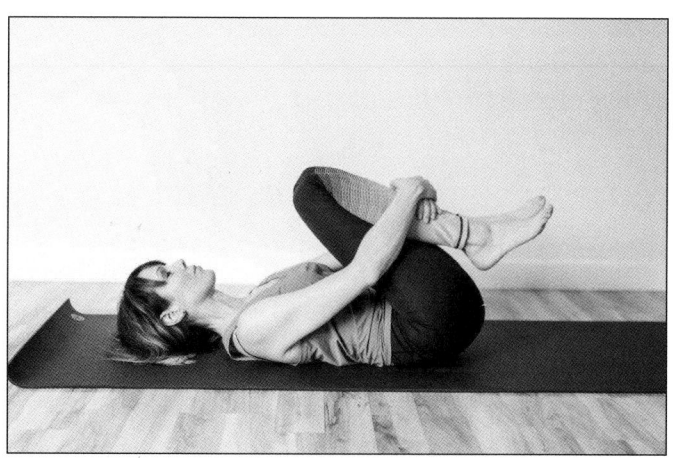

Tabletop–Thread the Needle

Start in tabletop with wrists underneath shoulders and knees underneath hips.

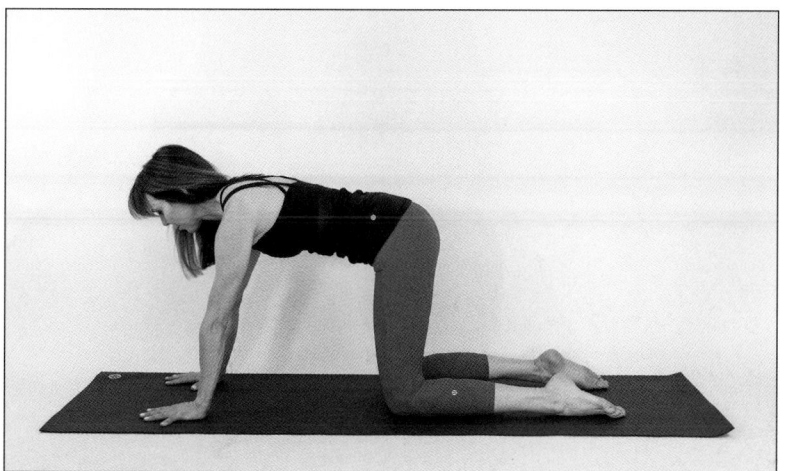

1. Inhale and reach your right arm up.

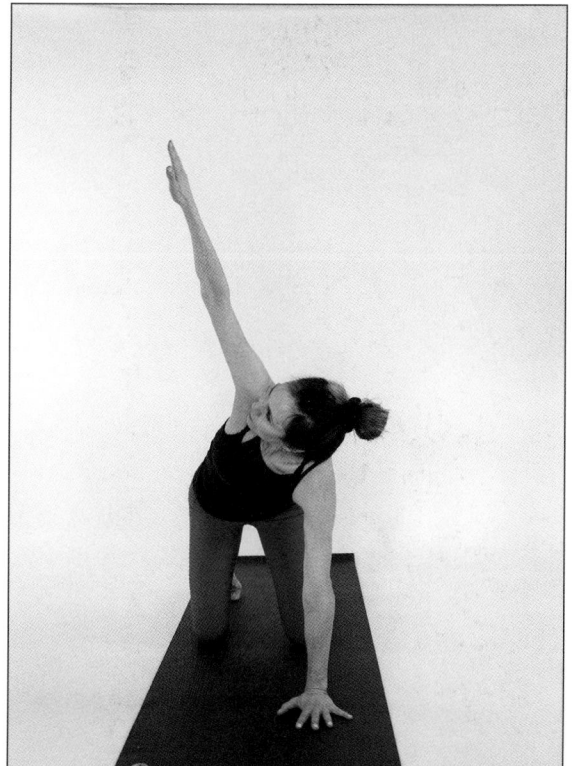

2. Exhale and thread your right arm under your left arm. Lower your right shoulder and ear to the ground. Keep equal weight in your knees, with feet straight out behind you.

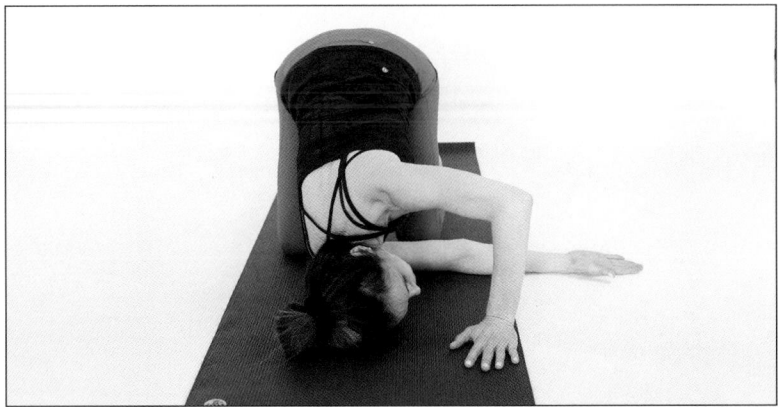

3. Hold for a few breaths and note how the pose feels in your body. Return to tabletop and repeat on other side

Reciprocal Reaching Stretch with Strap

1. Start seated on the floor with your legs tucked underneath you or in a chair. Drape a strap across your right shoulder (use an eight-foot strap or longer). Reach your right arm straight up and your left arm straight down alongside your body.
2. Bend both elbows so that your right palm and the back of your left hand both rest against your back. Hold the strap and crawl your fingers toward each other. Make sure your chin doesn't lift or lower too much. Keep your chin parallel with the floor and lengthen through the back of your neck.
3. Hold for several breaths and note how the pose feels in your body.
4. Release and repeat on the opposite side. Begin by draping the strap over your left shoulder.

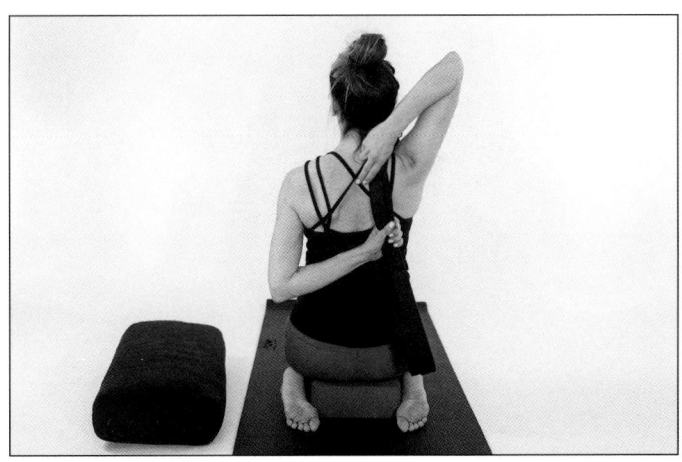

Mountain–Extended Mountain

1. Begin in mountain pose. Rotate the palms of both hands so that your thumbs point behind you and your palms are facing away from your thighs. Inhaling, reach your hands out and overhead so that your biceps face your ears.

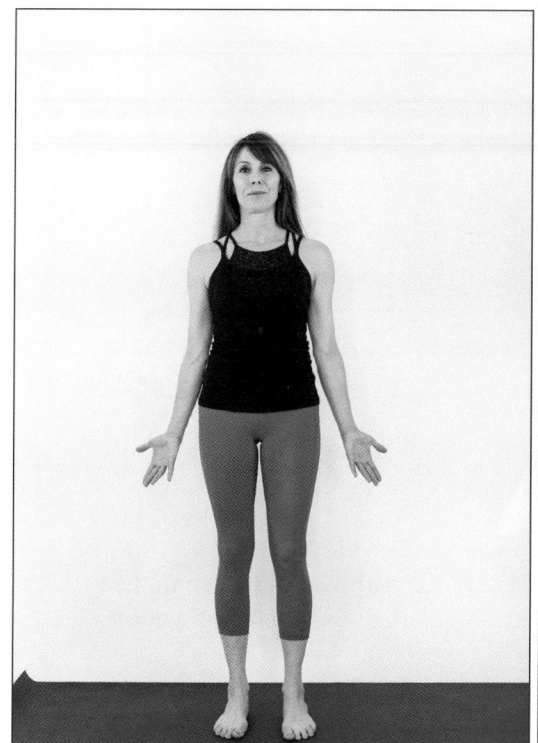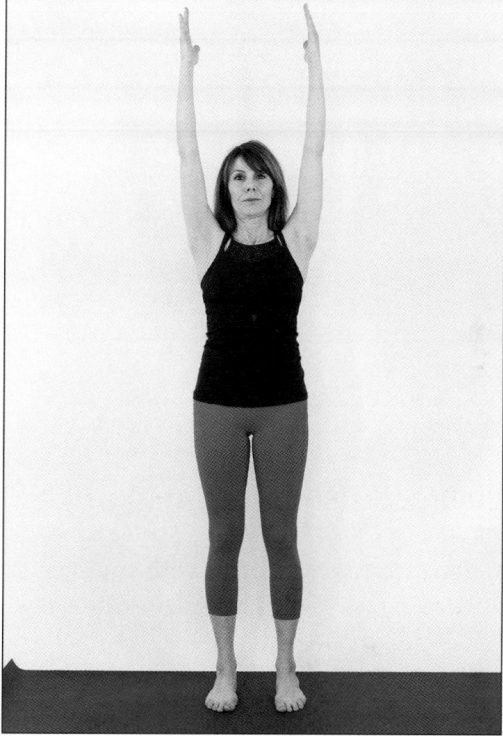

2. Soften the tops of your shoulders down. Hold for a few breaths, then release back into mountain pose.

Half Forward Fold

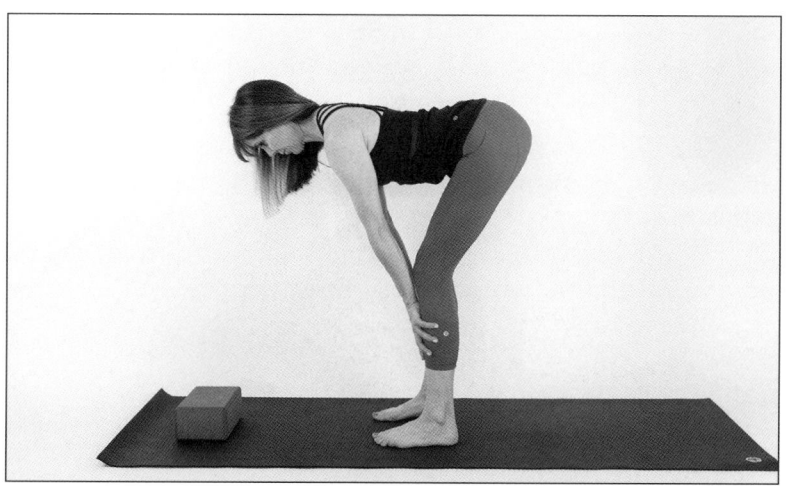

Child's

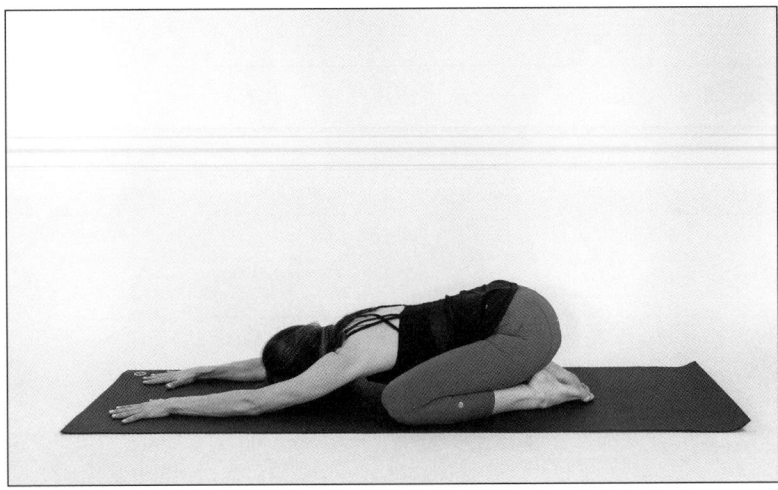

Savasana

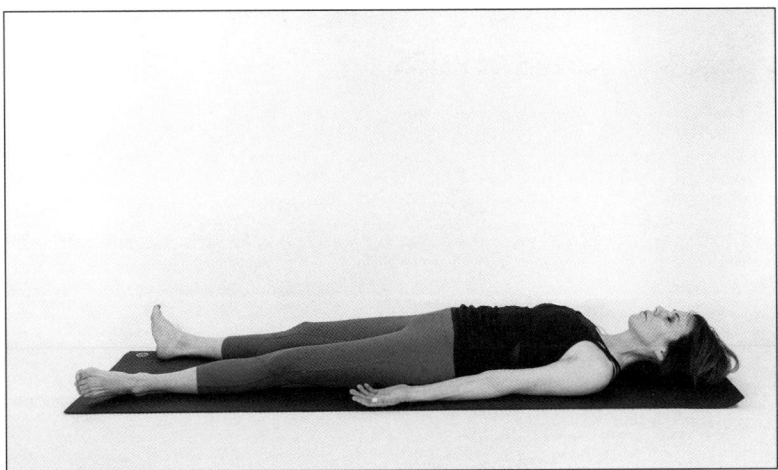

Week 3: Trunk Stability

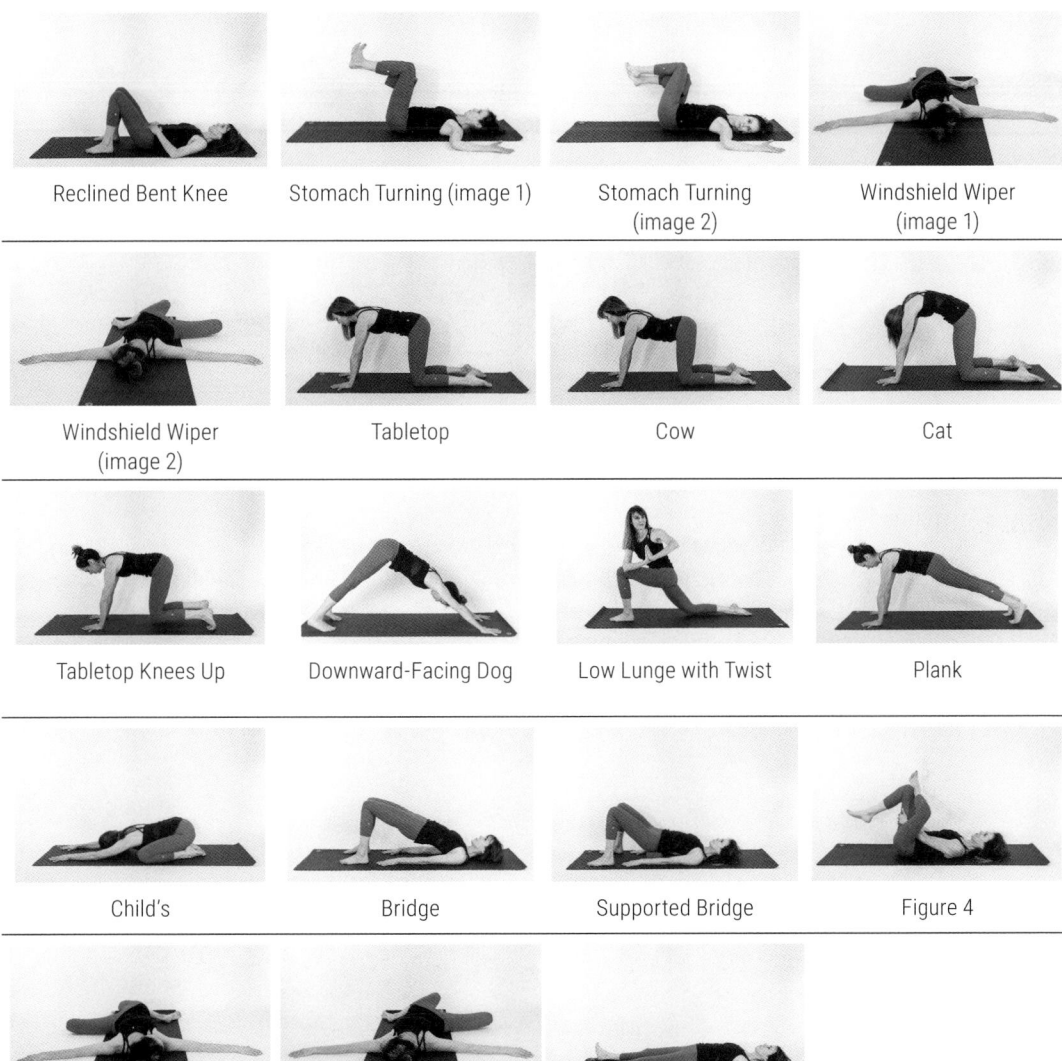

Reclined Bent Knee

Stomach Turning (image 1)

Stomach Turning (image 2)

Windshield Wiper (image 1)

Windshield Wiper (image 2)

Tabletop

Cow

Cat

Tabletop Knees Up

Downward-Facing Dog

Low Lunge with Twist

Plank

Child's

Bridge

Supported Bridge

Figure 4

Windshield Wiper (image 1)

Windshield Wiper (image 2)

Savasana

Reclined Bent Knee—Stomach Turning

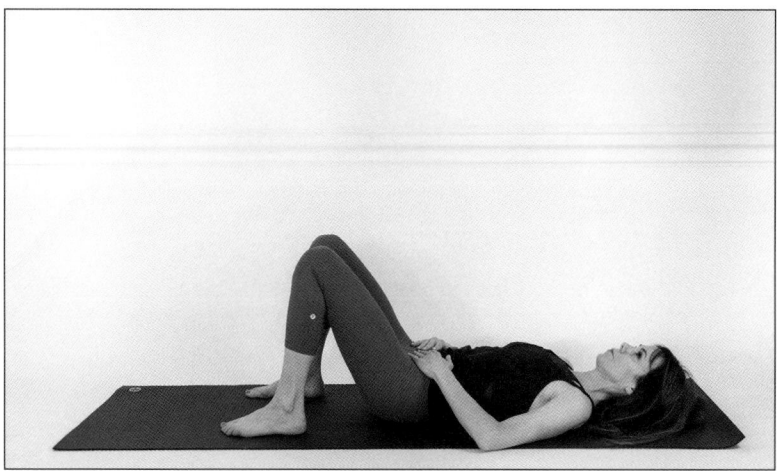

1. Start lying on your back with knees bent. Place a block or cushion between your thighs or above your knees. Alternatively, press your knees together.
2. Bend your elbows 90° (arms like a goalpost) and press the backs of your hands into the floor or, if it feels more comfortable, extend your arms out like a cross, and press your palms down.
3. Keeping your upper back and arms flush with the floor and lift your feet so that your knees stack over your hips and your calves are parallel with the floor.

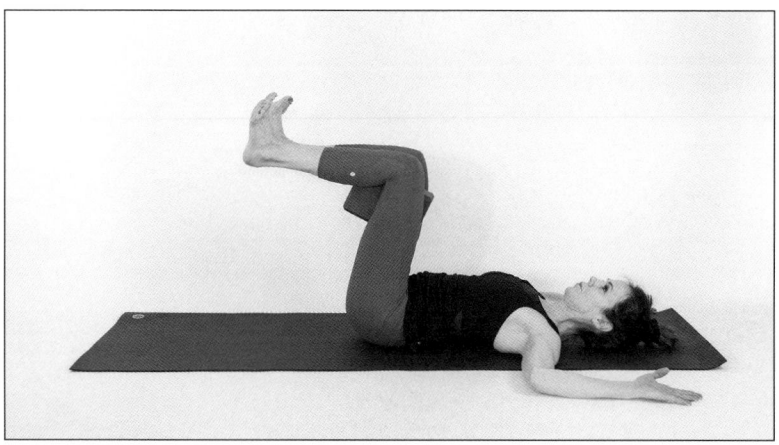

Flex your toes toward your shins. Begin rocking your knees gently from side to side to activate your core muscles.

4. On an inhalation, squeeze the block or press your thighs together to activate your inner legs, pelvic floor, and core. Lower your knees to the right while keeping your left shoulder and shoulder blade in contact with the floor. Gently rotate your head in the opposite direction. Exhaling, move your knees and head back to center.

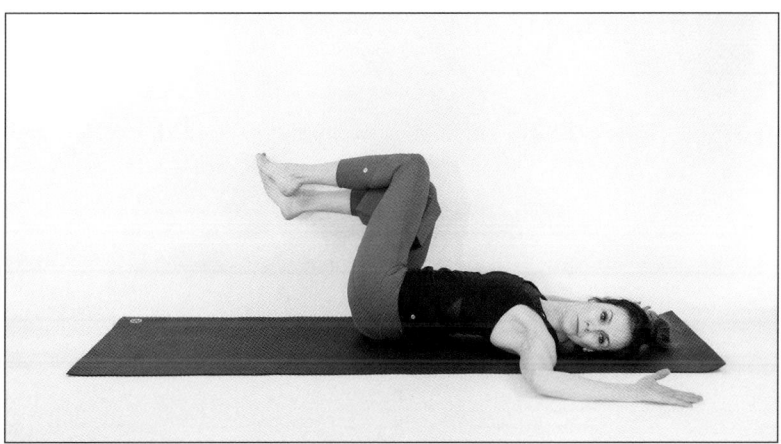

5. Inhaling, lower your knees to the left while keeping your right shoulder and shoulder blade in contact with the floor. Limit how far your knees lower if you feel a strain in your lower back. Gently rotate your head in the opposite direction relative to that in which your knees are lowering. Exhaling, move your knees back to center.
6. Practice the pose for several cycles of breath and note how it feels in your body.

Windshield Wiper

1. Start lying on your back. Bend your knees and slide your feet in a comfortable distance from your hips. Separate your feet wide enough that the outer edges of your feet line up with the edges of your mat. Move your arms away from your torso with palms up or down (your choice).
2. Lift your chest and draw your shoulder blades gently toward your spine. Lower both knees to the left and rotate your head to the right.

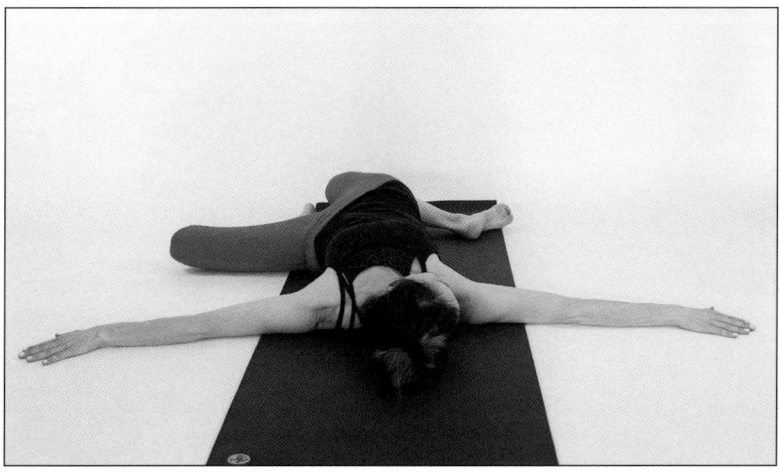

Then, revolve both knees to the right and rotate your head to left.

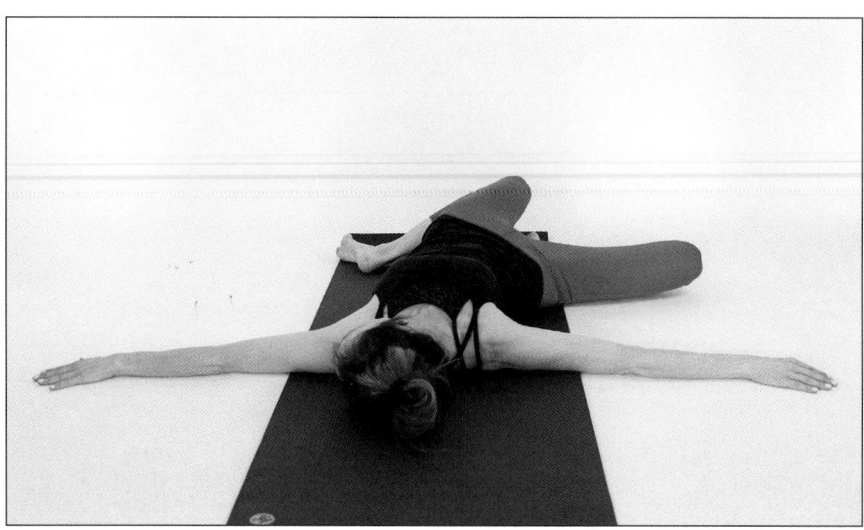

3.   Go back and forth several times, moving with your breath.

Tabletop

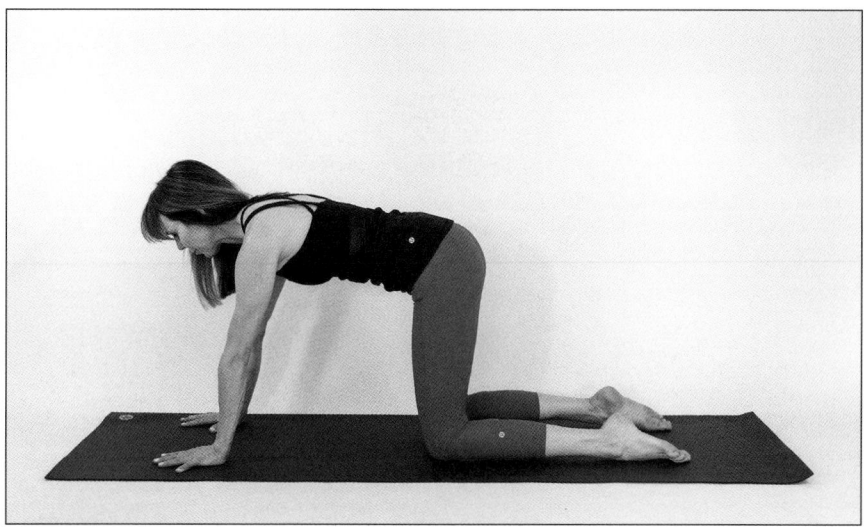

Cow

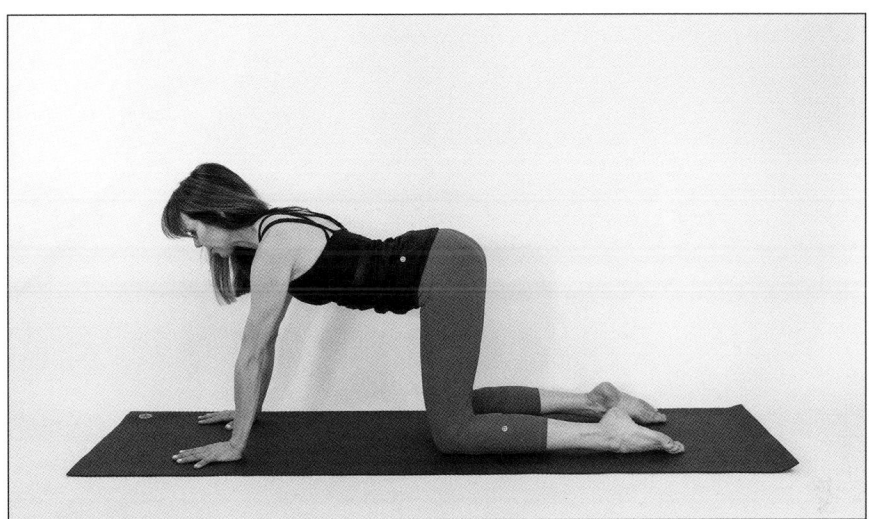

Cat

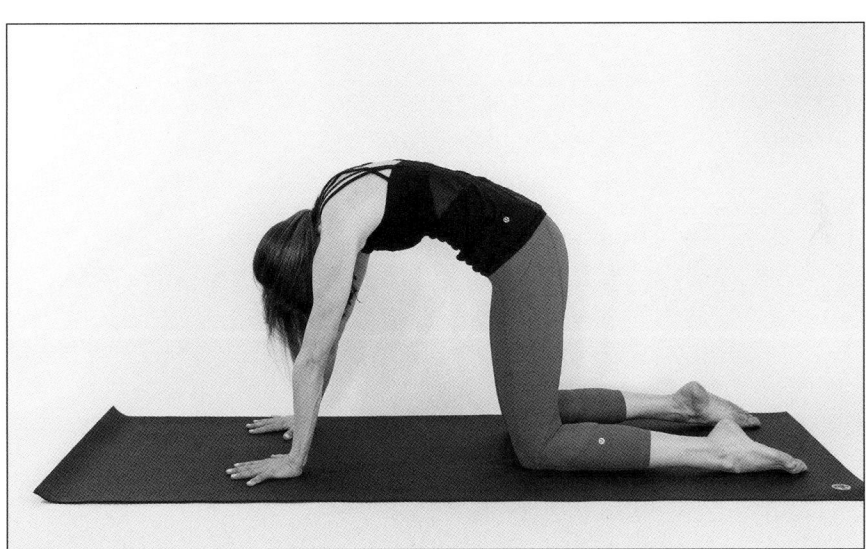

Tabletop Knees Up

1. Start in tabletop. Move your knees slightly closer to your wrists for stability. Tuck your toes and lift both knees off the ground about an inch. Let your knees hover as you hug your belly in and activate your core muscles.
2. Lower your knees to the ground to release.

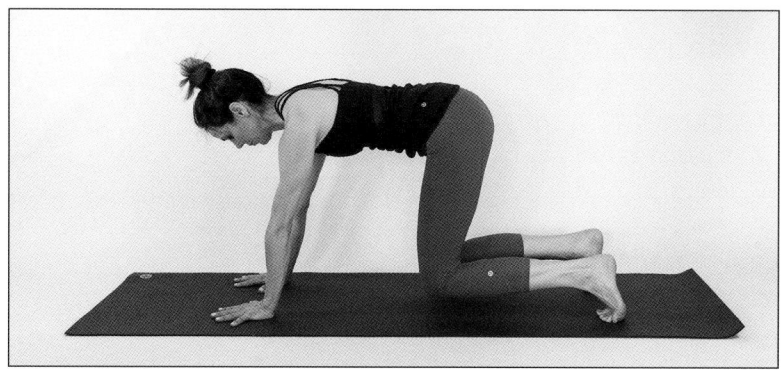

Downward-Facing Dog

1. Start in tabletop with wrists under shoulders and knees under hips. Bring your hands slightly forward relative to your shoulders, with your middle fingers pointing forward. Press firmly into your hands, anchoring down through the knuckle of your index finger on both hands. Spread your fingers to balance pressure in your wrists.
2. Begin to externally rotate and stabilize the shoulder joints by rolling your upper arms away from you. Draw your shoulders firmly against the back of your rib cage, creating more space across your upper back and allowing your neck to relax.
3. Tuck your toes under. On an exhalation, activate your lower belly, drawing your navel back to the spine.

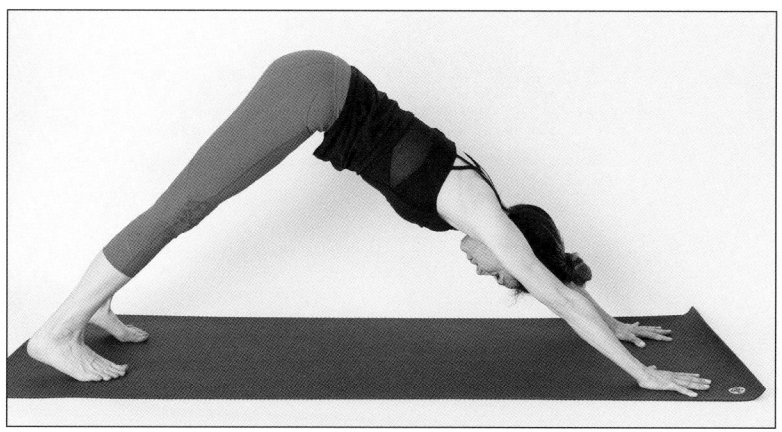

Press through your hands and lift your hips back and up to bring yourself into an upside-down **V** pose. Keep your knees bent at first as you find length in your spine.

4. Maintaining length in your spine, "walk your dog" by alternately bending and straightening your legs. Eventually try bringing both heels toward the floor. (They do not have to touch the floor.)
5. Hold for several breaths and note how the pose feels in your body.
6. To release, transition into child's pose.

Low Lunge with Twist

1. Start in low lunge with arms overhead. Release your right arm down and place that hand on your right hip.
2. Reach your left arm forward and across your body, twisting your torso toward your right thigh. Hook your left elbow on the outside of your right thigh. Press your palms together and turn your chest to the right.
3. Draw your right shoulder and shoulder blade back and down, looking down at your right foot to release the neck.
4. Hold for a few breaths and note how the pose feels in your body.
5. Release back into tabletop and repeat on the opposite side.

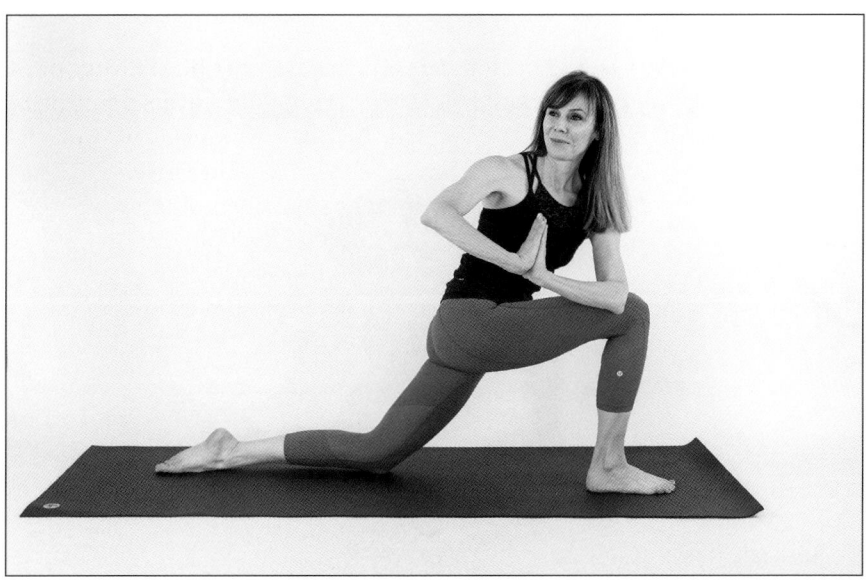

Plank

1. Start in tabletop. Step back with one foot and then the other, bringing your body into a push-up shape. Wiggle both feet back until your shoulders line up over your wrists. Pull the front of your rib cage in toward your spine and draw your shoulders down and away from your ears. Don't let your plank sag!
2. Extend your heels back and the crown of your head forward, lengthening your entire body. Keep your gaze forward and down to allow your neck to naturally extend from your spine.
3. Hold for a few breaths and lower your knees into tabletop.

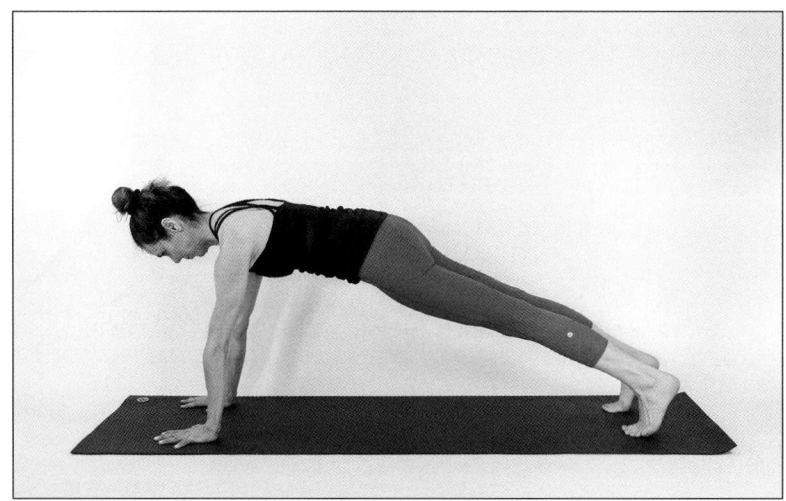

Child's

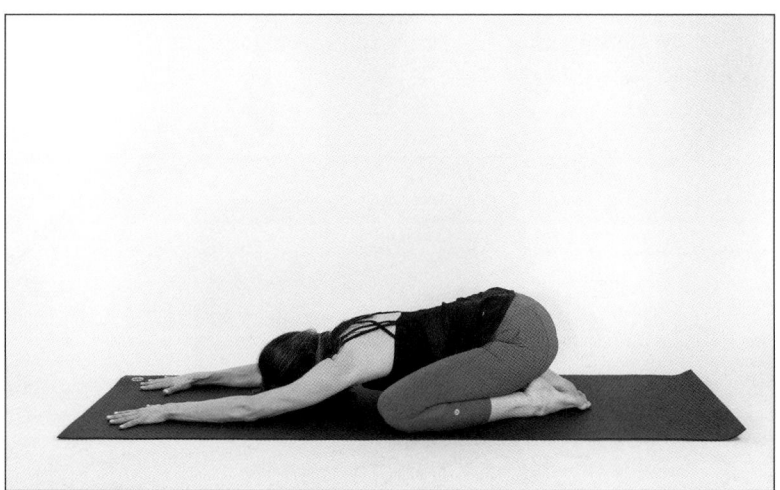

Bridge

1. Start on your back with your knees bent and feet hip-width apart. Rest your arms on the floor near your hips with palms facing down. Press down through both feet and lift your hips up until they are level with your knees.
2. Keeping your knees in line with your hips, draw your inner thighs down toward the floor.
3. Draw your shoulder blades down your back and relax your face and jaw.
4. Hold for a few breaths and then release your hips down to the floor.

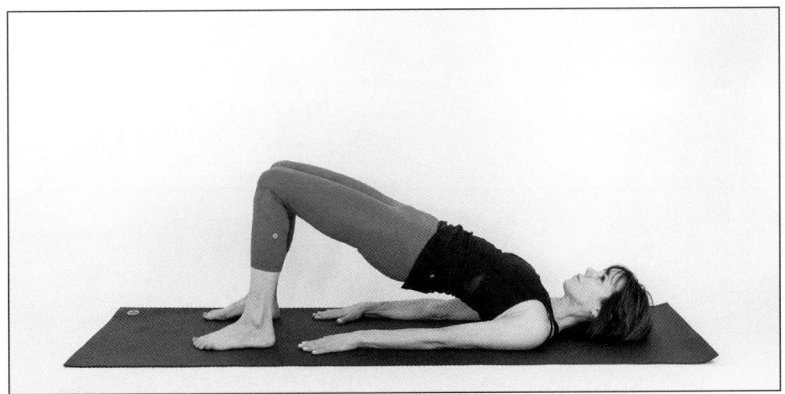

Supported Bridge

1. Start in bridge. Place a yoga block or bolster under your sacrum (not your lower back). Rest the weight of your lower body on the block to passively arch your lower spine and open the front of your pelvis.
2. Be mindful of your breathing.
3. To release, lift your hips up and slide the support out from underneath you, then slowly roll your spine back down to the mat.

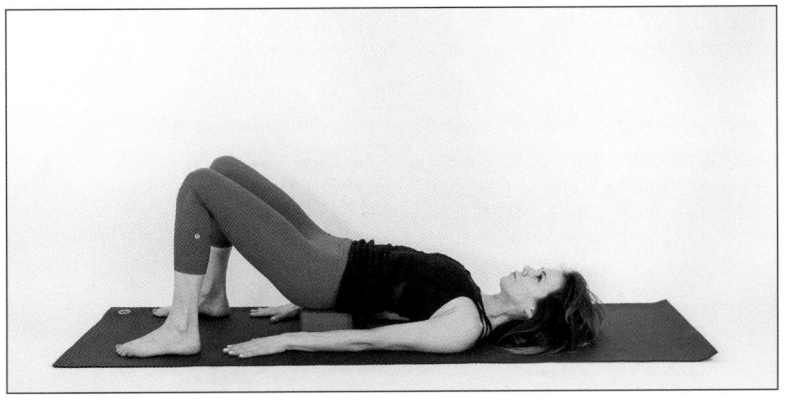

Figure 4

1. Start lying on your back. Bend your knees and slide your feet in close to your buttocks, hip-distance apart and parallel.
2. Cross the outer aspect of your right ankle over your left thigh, allowing your right knee to move away from your right armpit. Reach both hands around and clasp your left thigh (unless this causes your upper back or head to lift, in which case let go and rest your arms on the floor). Gently pull your left knee toward your chest.
3. Hold for several breaths and note how the pose feels in your body.
4. Release your right foot back to the floor and repeat on the opposite side.

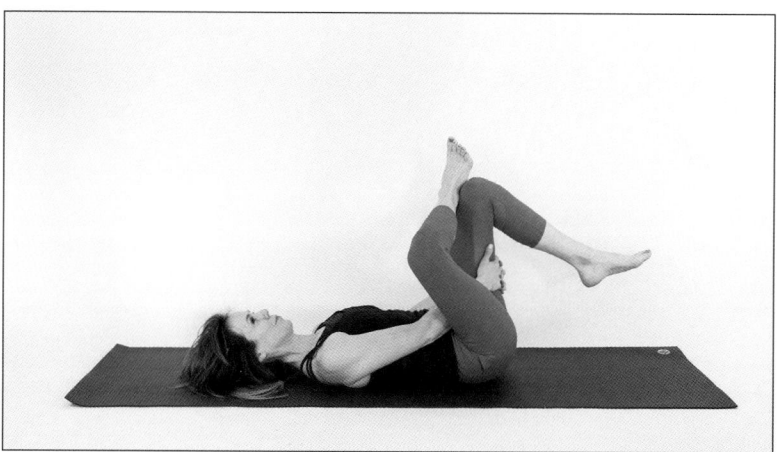

Windshield Wiper

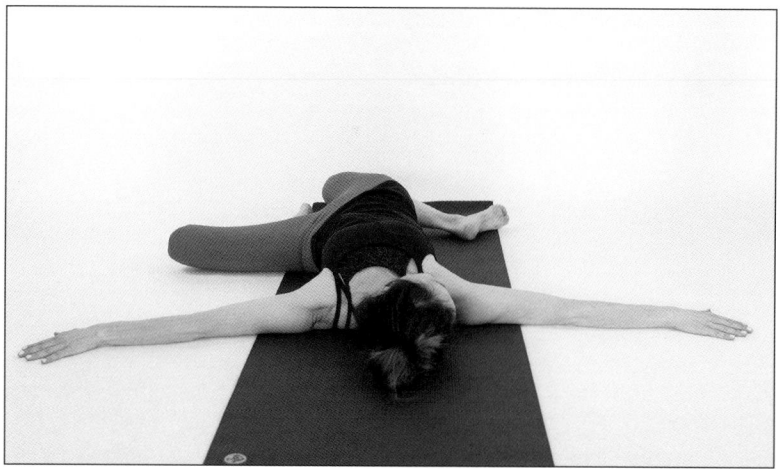

Windshield Wiper (continued)

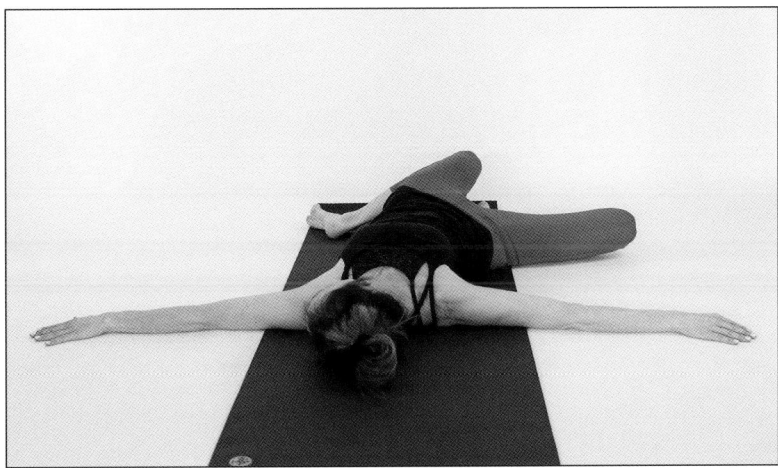

Savasana

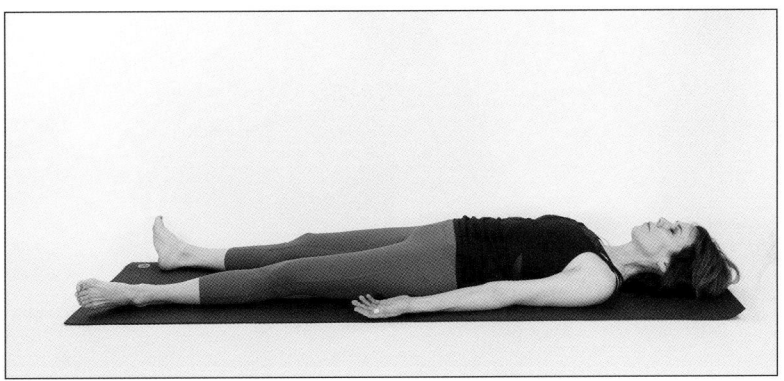

Week 4: The Balancing Act

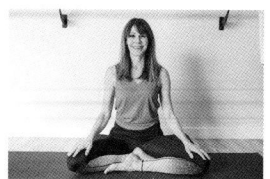

Simple Cross-Legged Seat

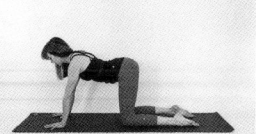

Cow

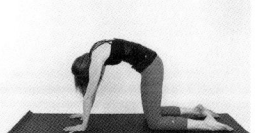

Cat

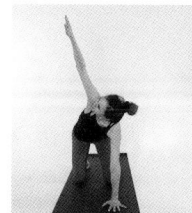

Thread the Needle
(image 1)

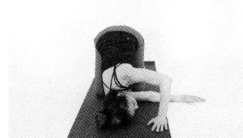

Thread the Needle
(image 2)

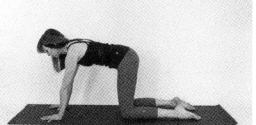

Tabletop

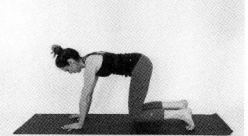

Tabletop Knees Up

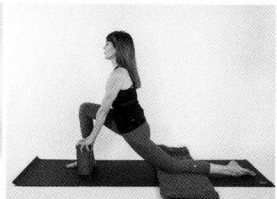

Low Lunge with Props

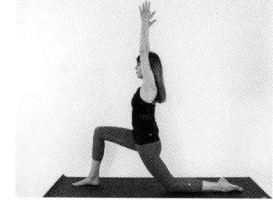

Low Lunge

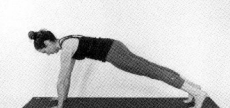

Plank

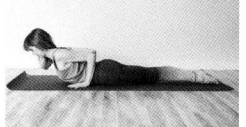

Locust

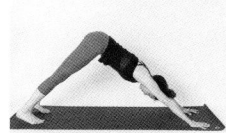

Downward Facing Dog

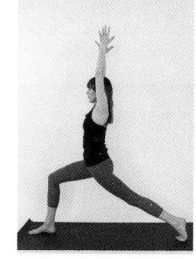

Crescent Lunge

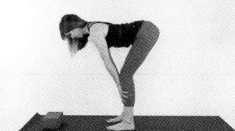

Half Forward Fold

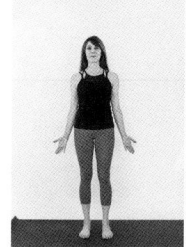

Mountain

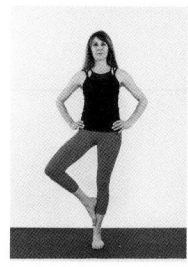

Tree

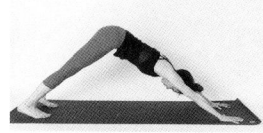

Downward-Facing Dog

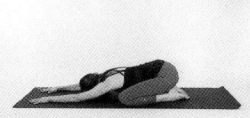

Child's

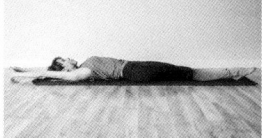

Full-Body Stretch

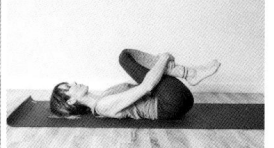

Upward-Facing Child's

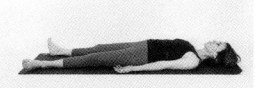

Savasana

Simple Cross-Legged Seat

1. Start sitting cross-legged on the floor. If your knees are higher than your hips, try sitting on a yoga block or firm bolster to get your hips above your knees, allowing your pelvis to rotate toward the lumbar spine and preventing you from tipping back.

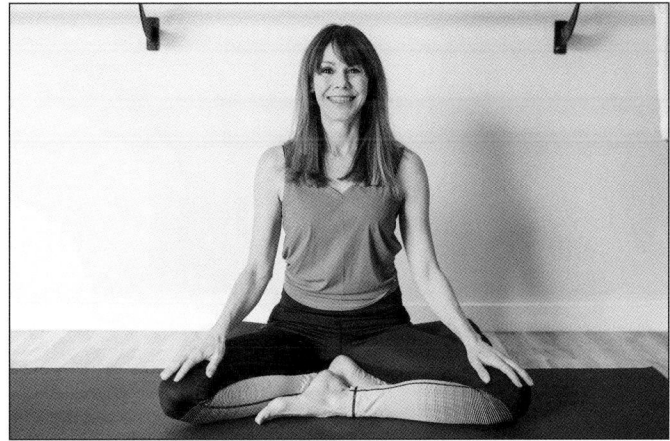

2. Press down through your pelvis and lift through your torso, with shoulder blades pressing down against the back of the rib cage.
3. Let your palms rest on your thighs.
4. Hold for several breaths and note how the pose feels in your body.

Cow

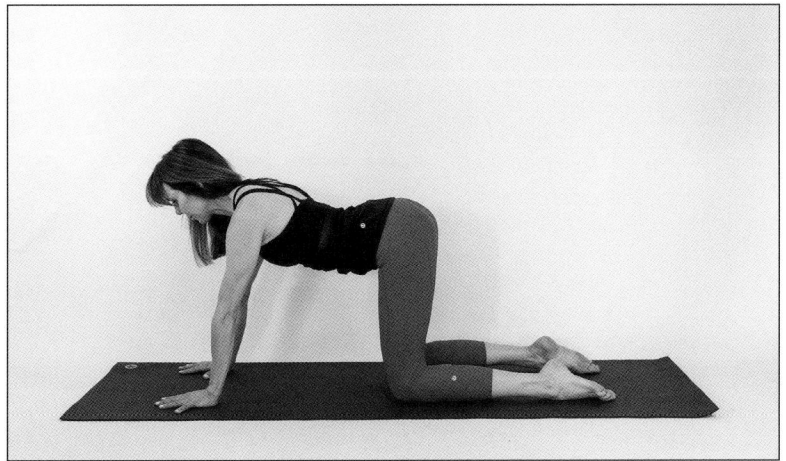

Cat

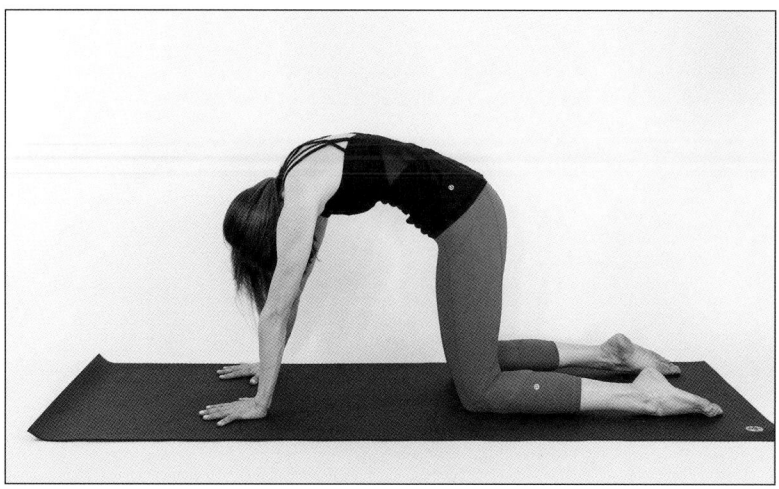

Thread the Needle

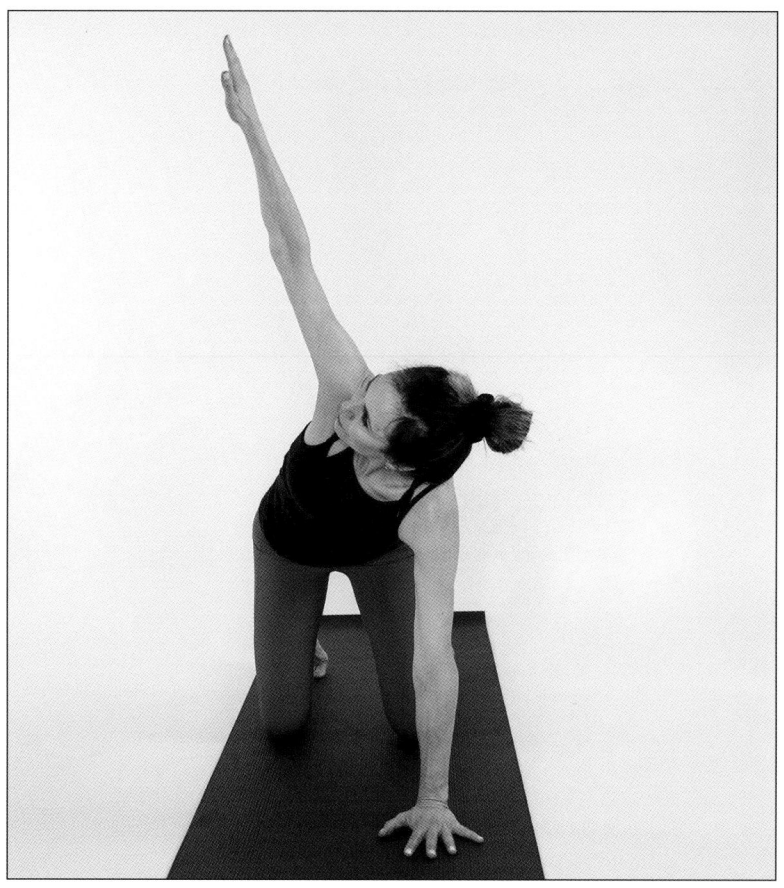

Thread the Needle (continued)

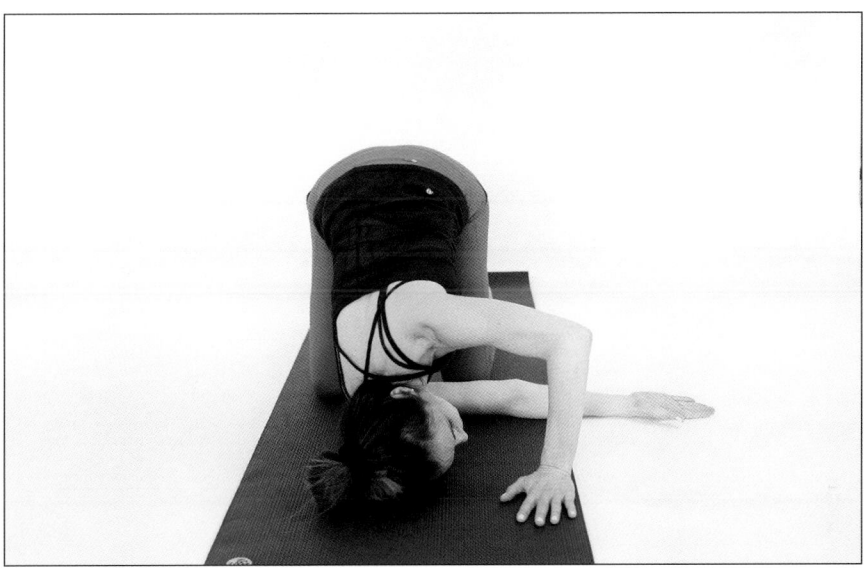

Tabletop

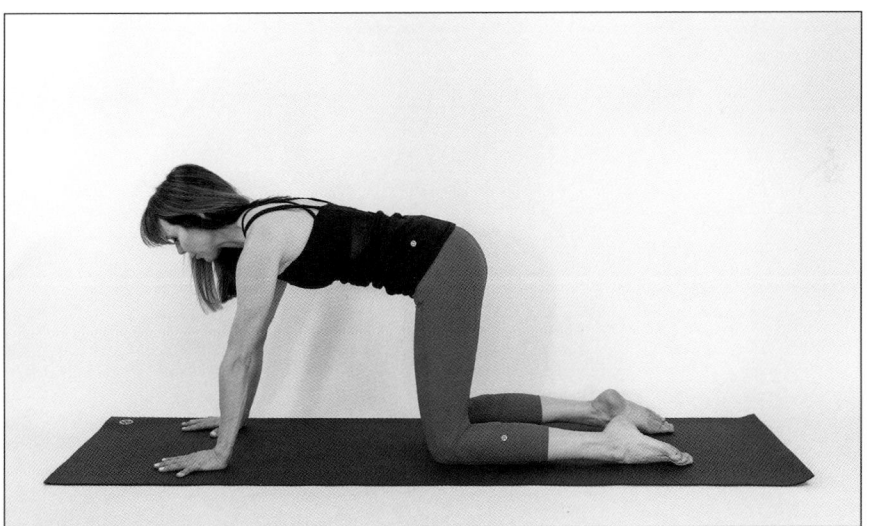

Tabletop Knees Up

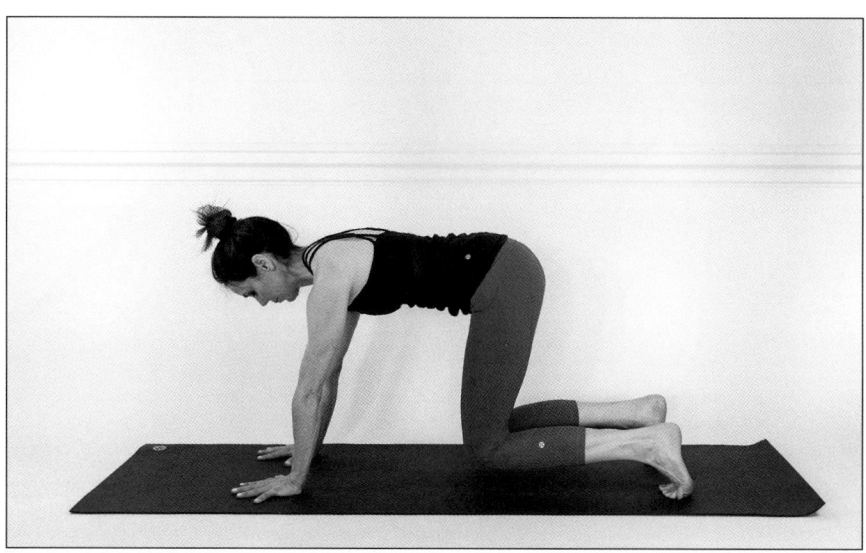

Low Lunge—Low Lunge with Props

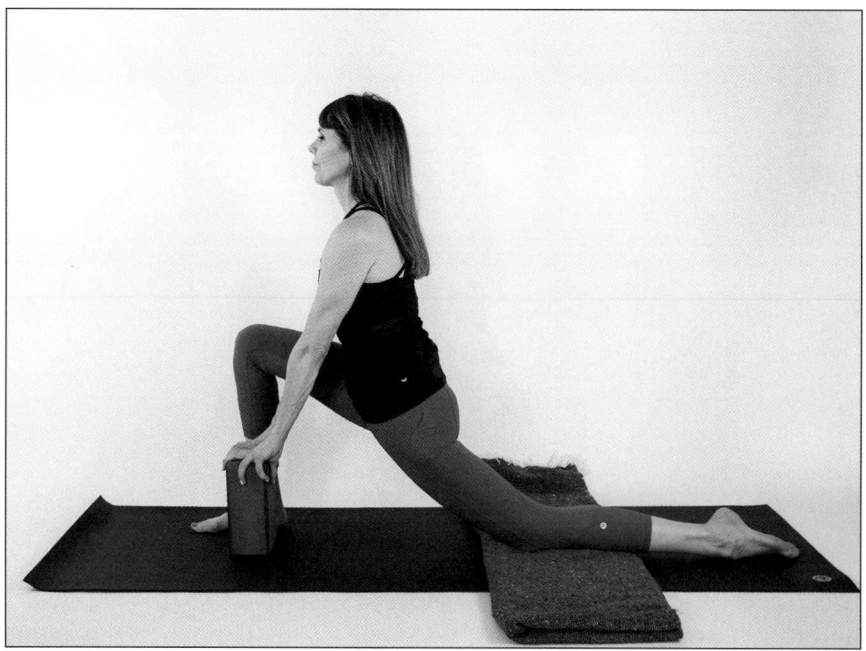

Low Lunge–Low Lunge with Props (continued)

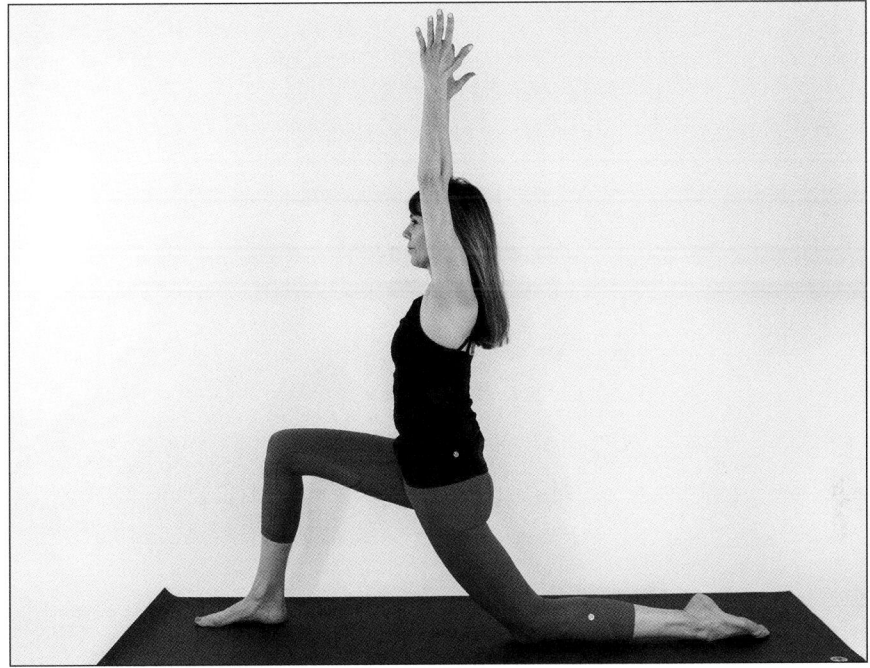

Plank

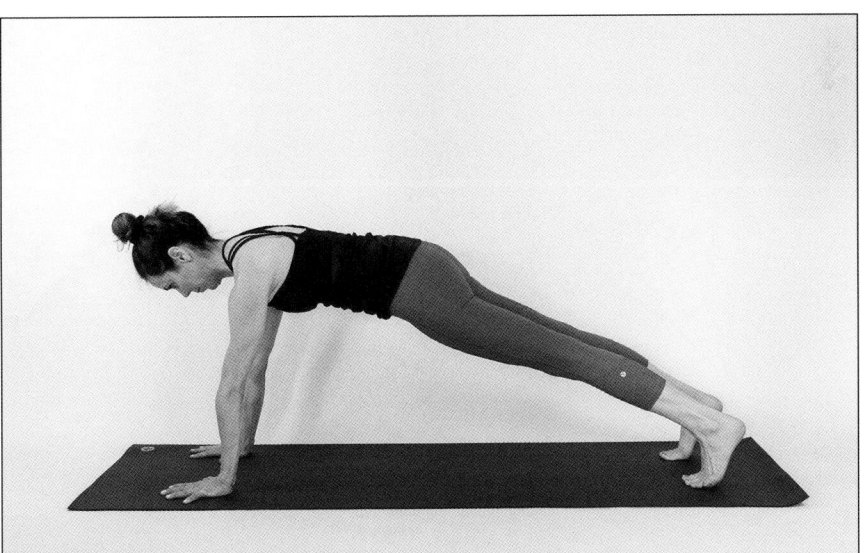

Locust

1. Start in a push-up position (plank pose). Lower your knees to the floor, then lower your abdomen, chest, and forehead to the floor at the same time.
2. Extend both legs behind you and angle your tailbone toward your heels. Slide your palms away from your shoulders and toward the middle of your rib cage, feeling the front of your shoulders gently lift away from the floor.
3. Press your hips and feet firmly into the floor. Begin lifting your forehead, shoulder, and chest, using your back and lower body strength, not arm strength.
4. Hold for a few breaths and release by lowering your chest, shoulders, and forehead.

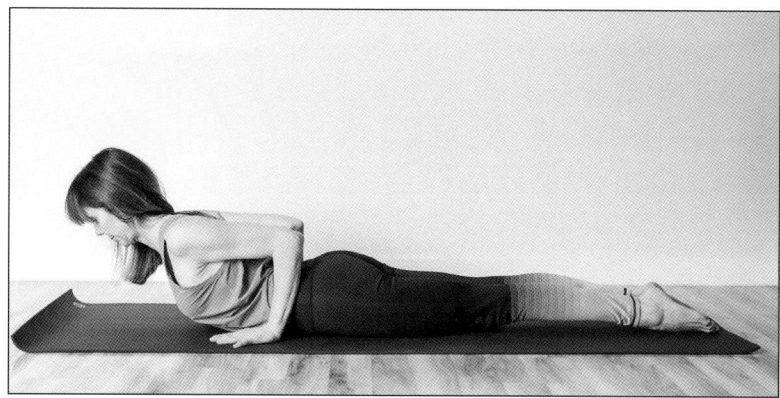

Downward-Facing Dog—Crescent Lunge

1. Start in downward-facing dog. Step your right foot between your hands and stack right knee over right ankle. Lift your torso upright to stack shoulders over hips. Your torso and the front of your pelvis are perpendicular to the floor. Soften the back knee to angle your tailbone down.

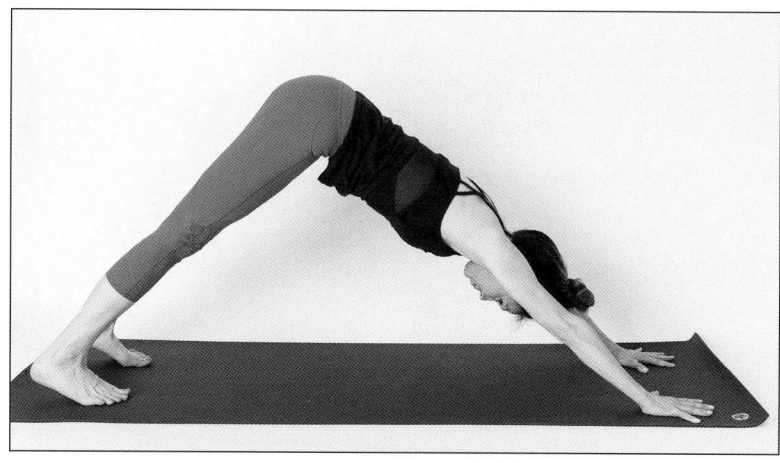

2.   Place your hands on your hips to level your pelvis. Maintaining a neutral pelvis, release your arms down by your sides. Turn your palms out to externally rotate and stabilize your shoulder joints and reach your arms out and overhead.

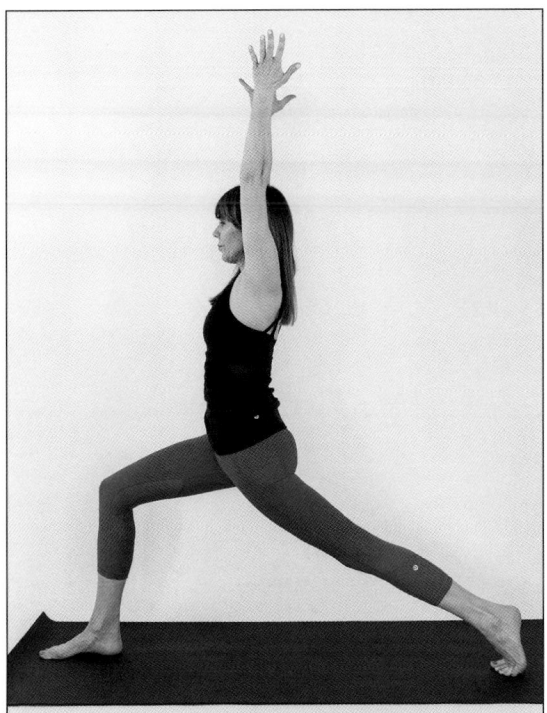

3.   To release, bring both hands to your hips and then to the floor. Step back into downward-facing dog and repeat on the other side.

Half Forward Fold

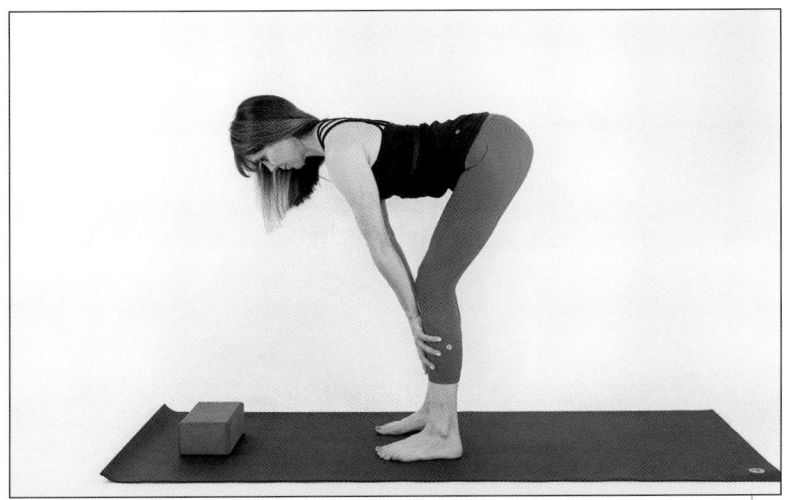

Mountain–Tree

1. Start in mountain, standing tall. Shift your weight to your right leg and bring your left foot onto the inside of your right calf. Focus your gaze at eye level or on the floor.

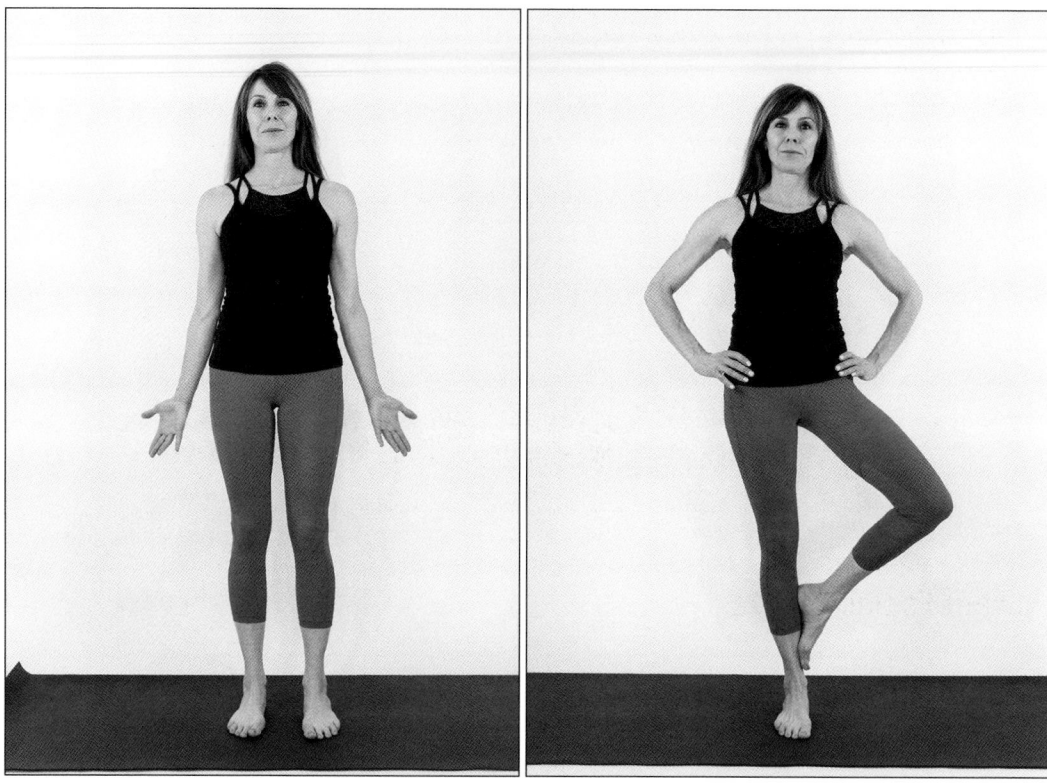

2. Slowly slide your left foot up your inner right shin just below or above your knee. Hold for a few breaths and feel the pose in your body.
3. Release back into mountain pose. Repeat on the opposite side.

Child's

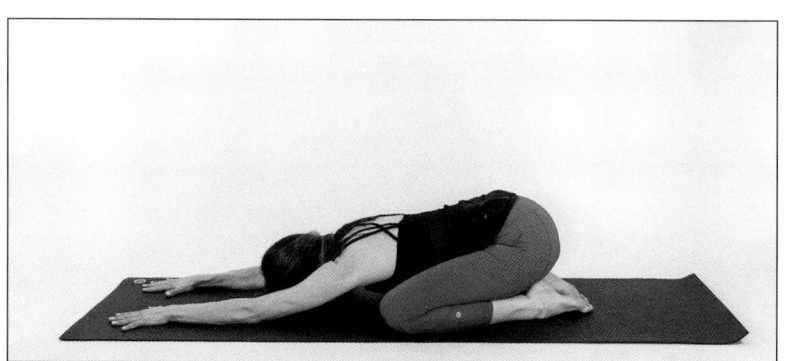

Full-Body Stretch

1. Start lying on your back, extending your legs on the floor. Draw your legs together and point your toes away from your shins.
2. Lift your arms overhead, interlace your fingers, and press your palms behind you. Flatten the front of your rib cage toward the floor to decrease the arch in your lower back.
3. Draw a deep breath in, stretch your entire body, exhale, and release your arms alongside your body and soften your legs. Note how the pose feels in your body.

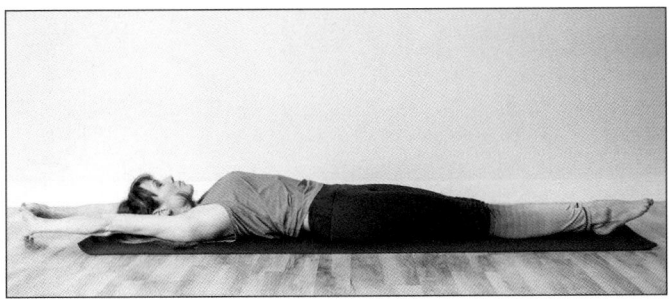

Upward-Facing Child's

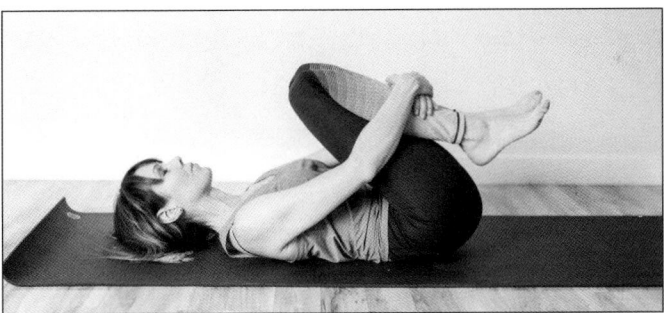

Savasana

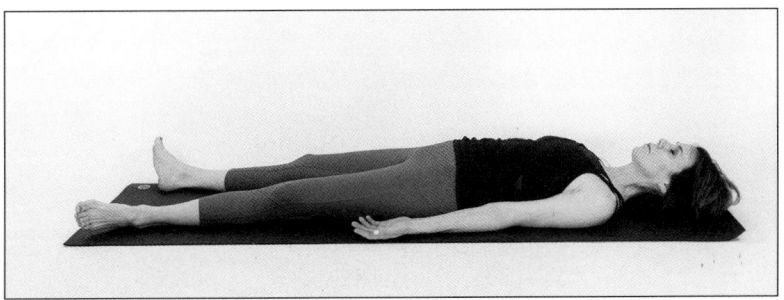

Week 5: #ItAllConnects

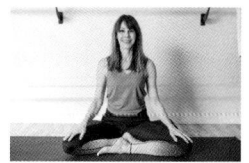

Simple Cross-Legged Seat

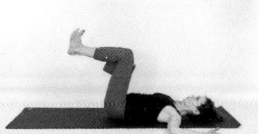

Stomach Turning
(image 1)

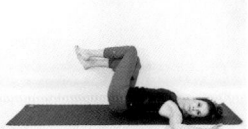

Stomach Turning
(image 2)

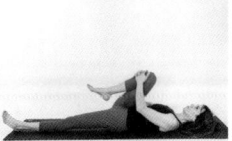

Reclined Single
Knee to Chest

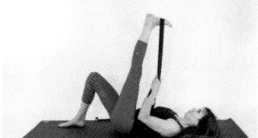

Reclined Big Toe
(image 1)

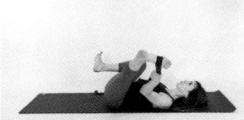

Reclined Big Toe
(image 2)

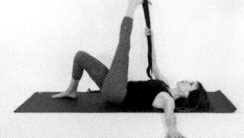

Reclined Big Toe
(image 3)

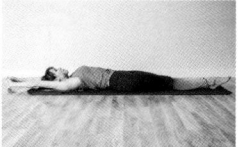

Full-Body Stretch

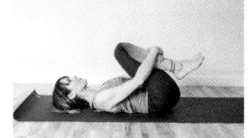

Upward-Facing Child's

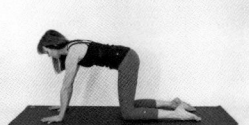

Tabletop

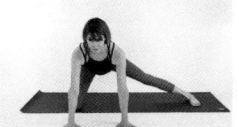

Gate Latch

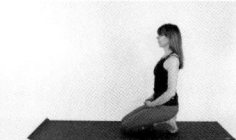

Toe Stretch

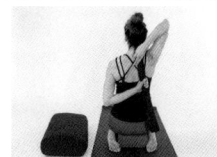

Reciprocal Reaching
Stretch with Strap

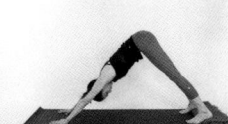

Downward-Facing
Dog Heels Up

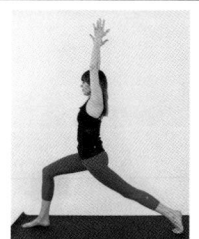

Crescent Lunge

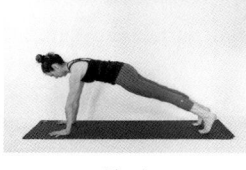

Plank

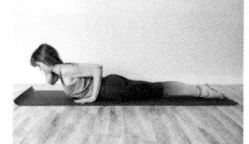

Locust

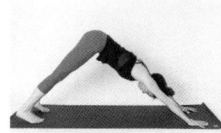

Downward-Facing Dog

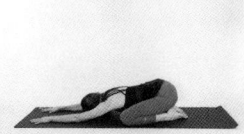

Child's

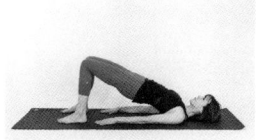

Bridge

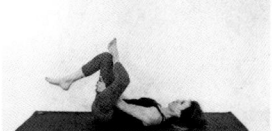

Figure 4

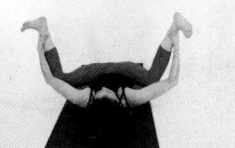

Happy Baby

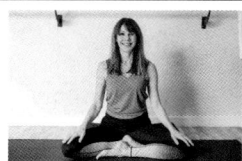

Simple Cross-Legged Seat

Simple Cross-Legged Seat

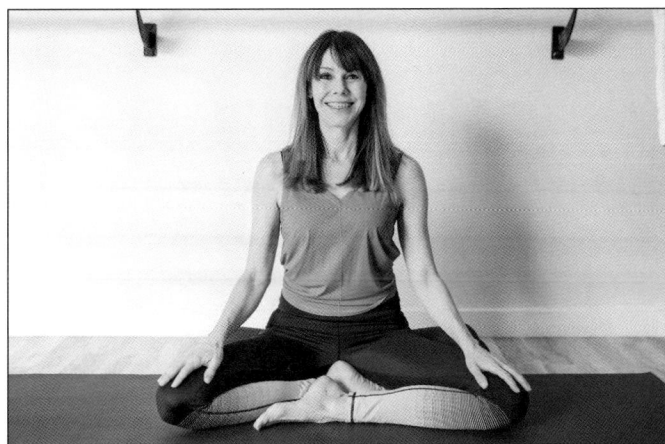

Stomach Turning

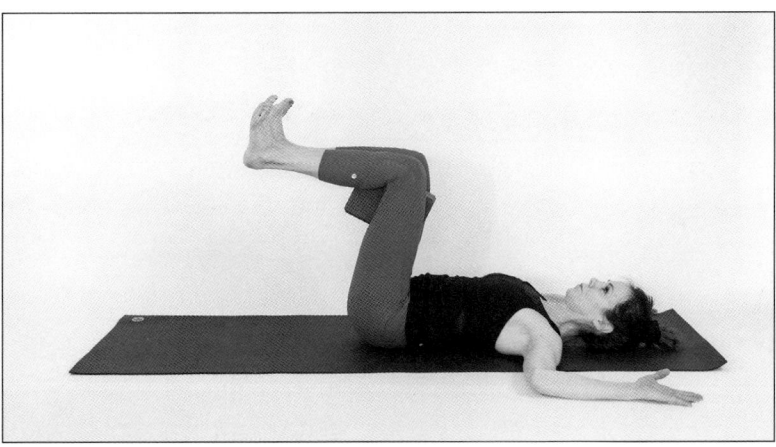

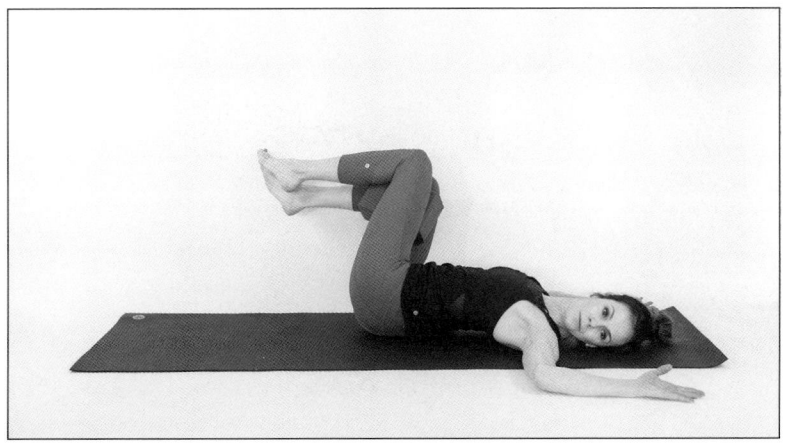

Reclined Single Knee to Chest

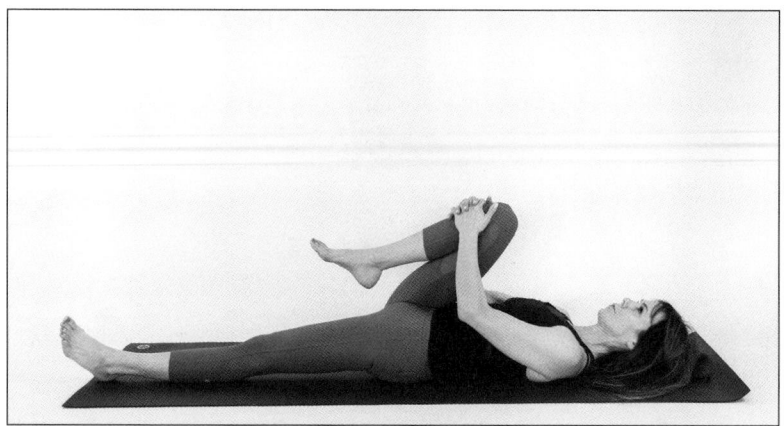

Reclined Big Toe

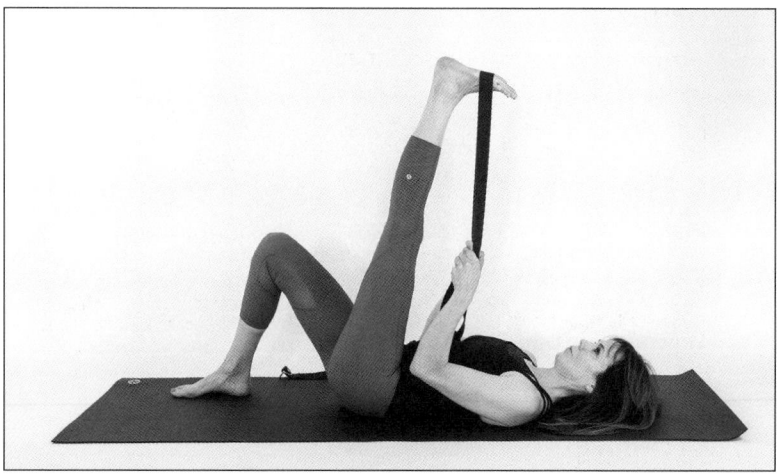

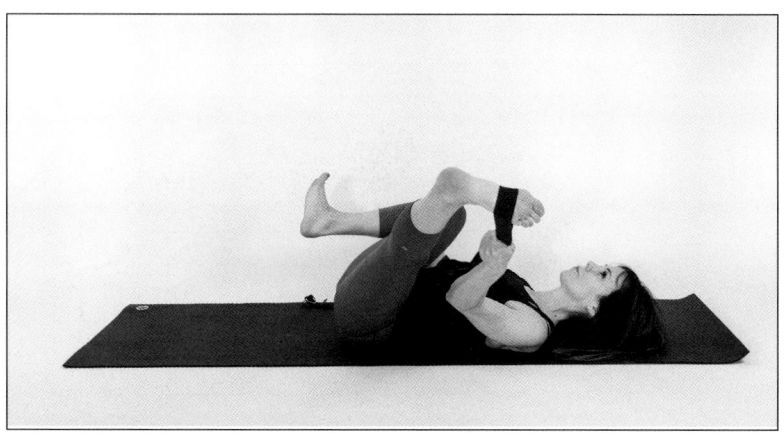

Reclined Big Toe (continued)

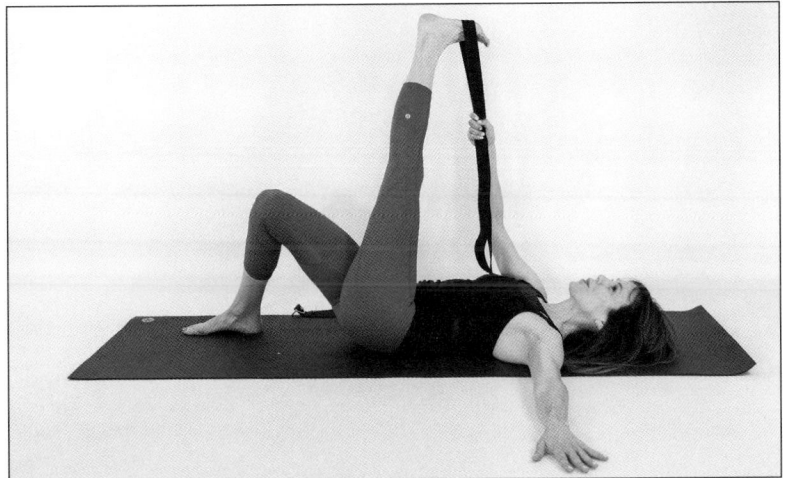

Full-Body Stretch

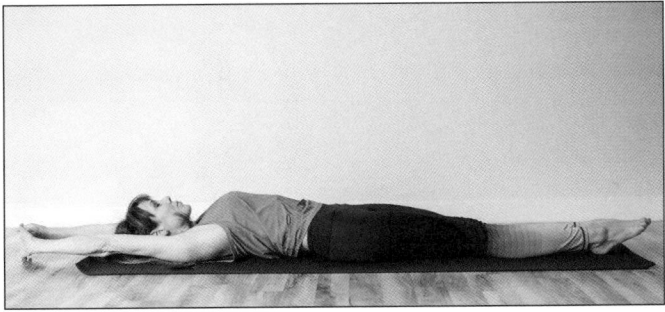

Upward-Facing Child's

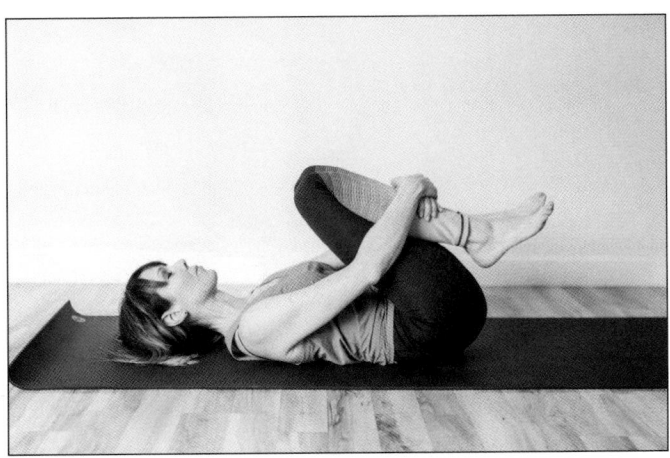

Tabletop–Gate Latch–Toe Stretch

1. Start in tabletop with wrists underneath shoulders and knees underneath hips.

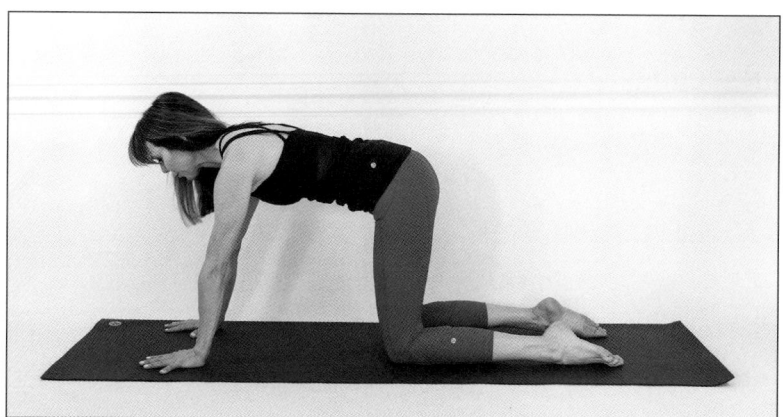

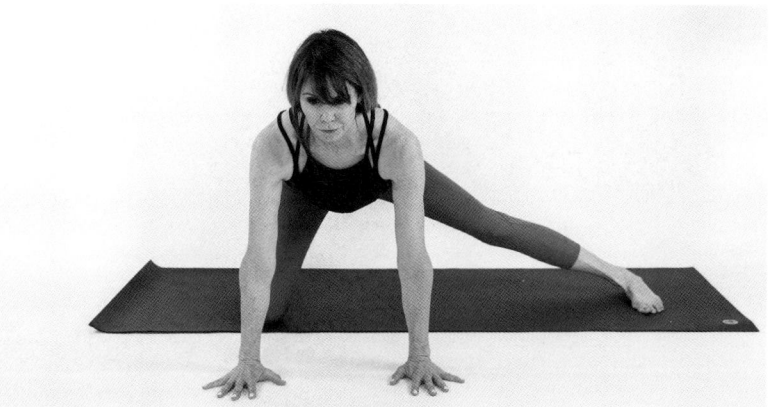

Tuck your toes and release your hips slowly back toward your heels.

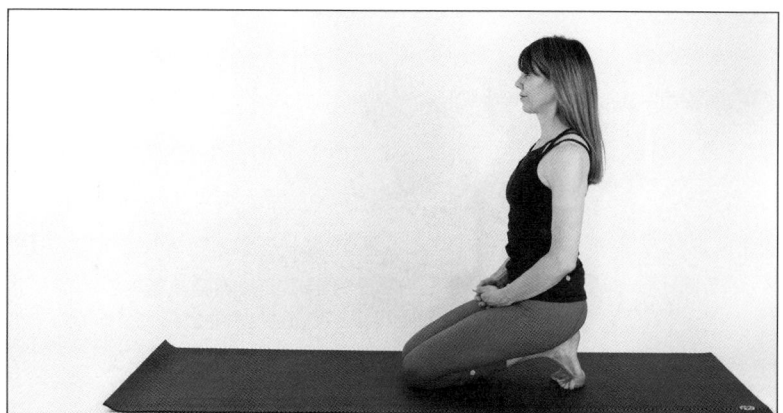

2.   You can adjust the pressure in your feet by keeping your palms or fingertips on the ground. Pay attention to the pressure in your toes and the soles of your feet.
3.   Lift your chest upright to sit on your heels, stacking shoulders over hips and resting palms on thighs.
4.   Hold for a few breaths and note how the pose feels in your body.

Reciprocal Reaching Stretch with Strap

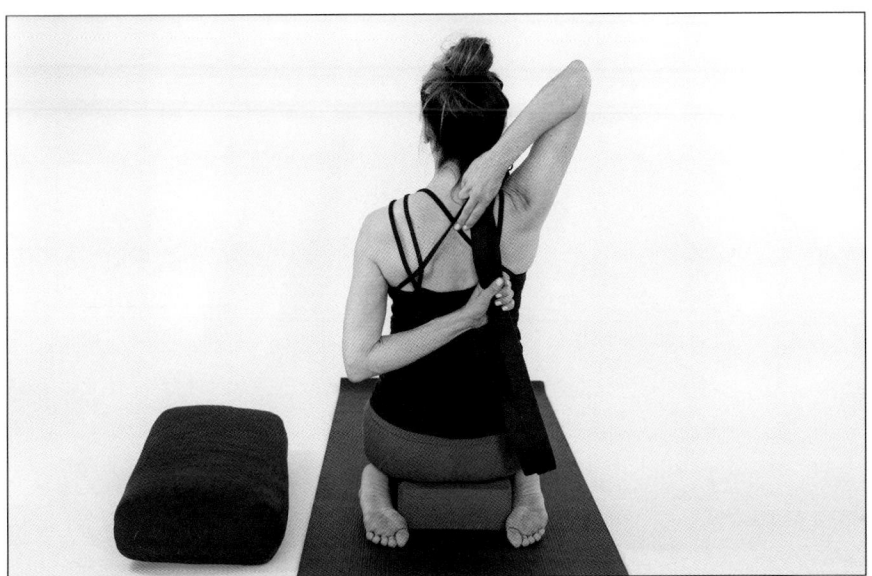

Downward-Facing Dog Heels Up

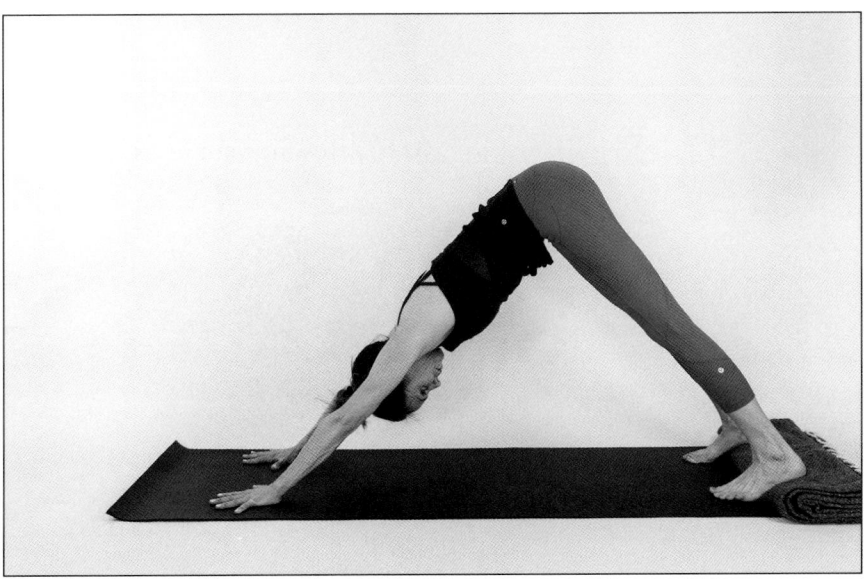

Crescent Lunge

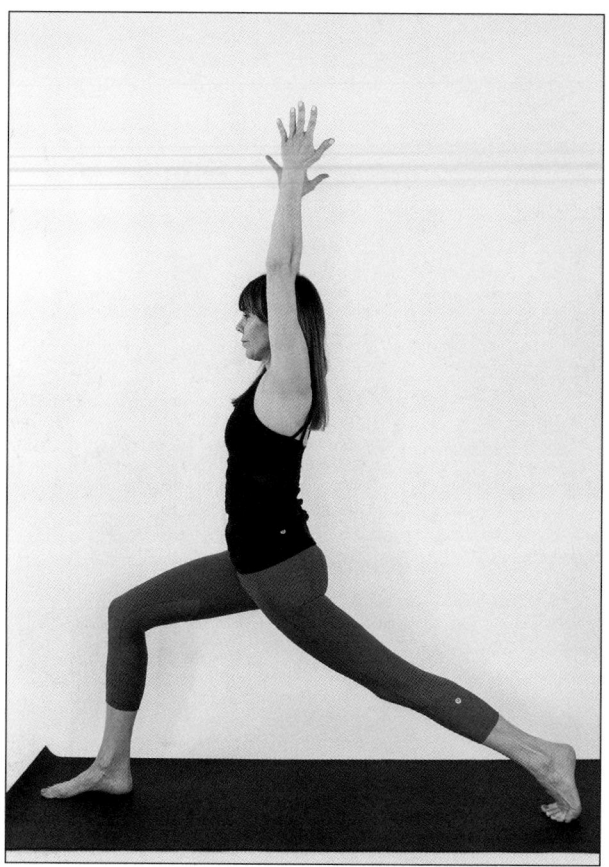

Plank

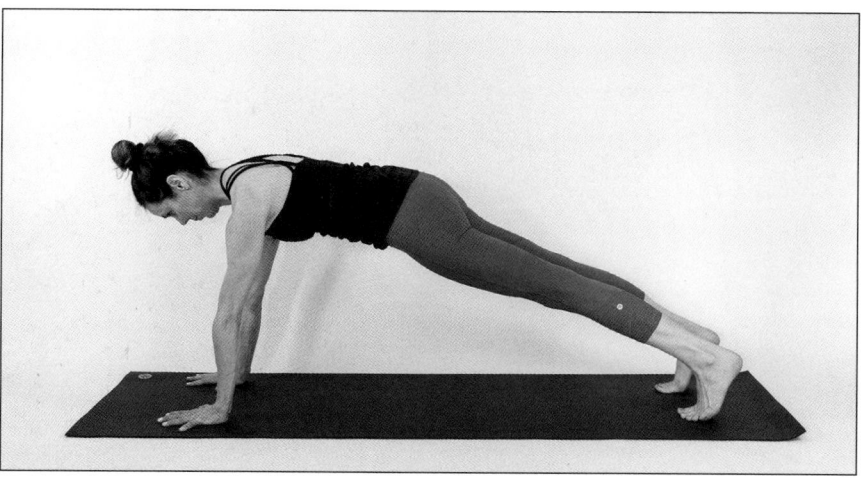

Locust

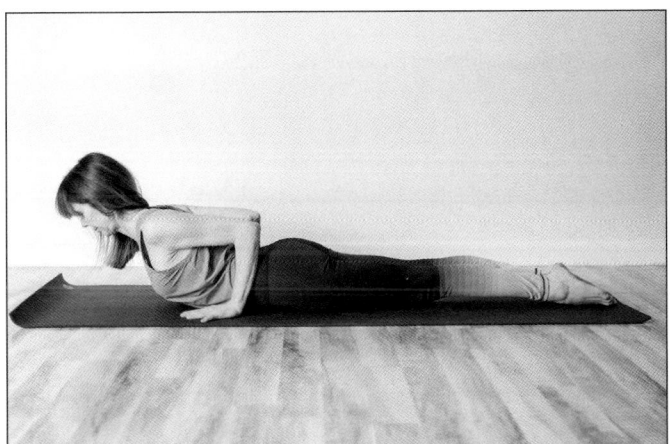

Downward-Facing Dog

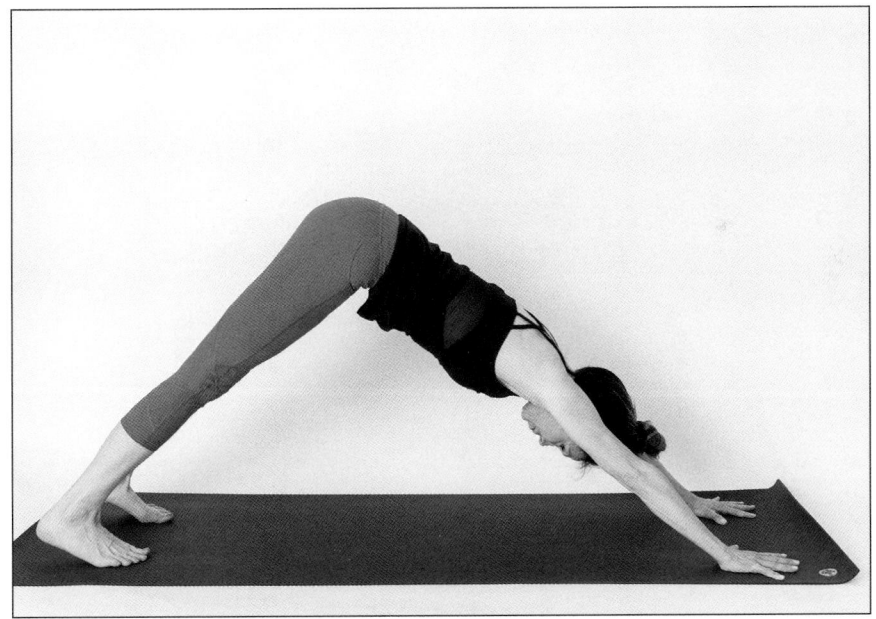

Child's

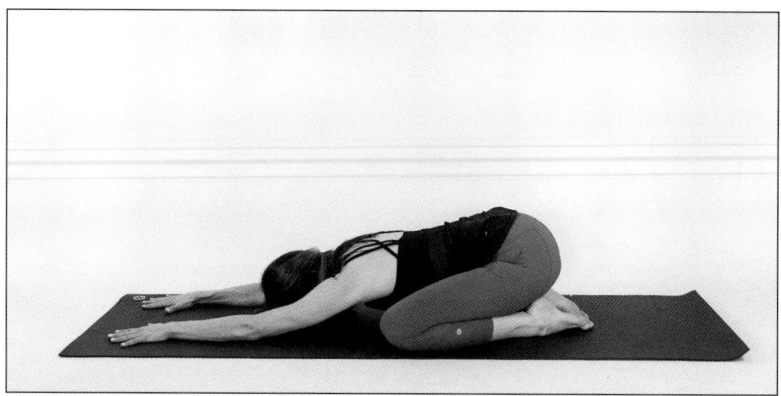

Bridge

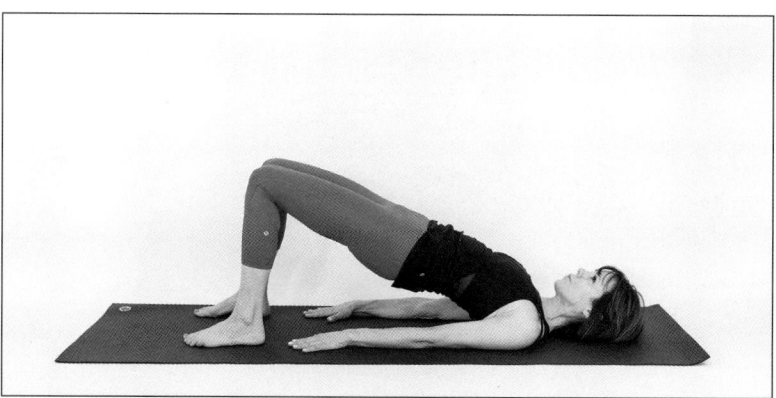

Figure 4

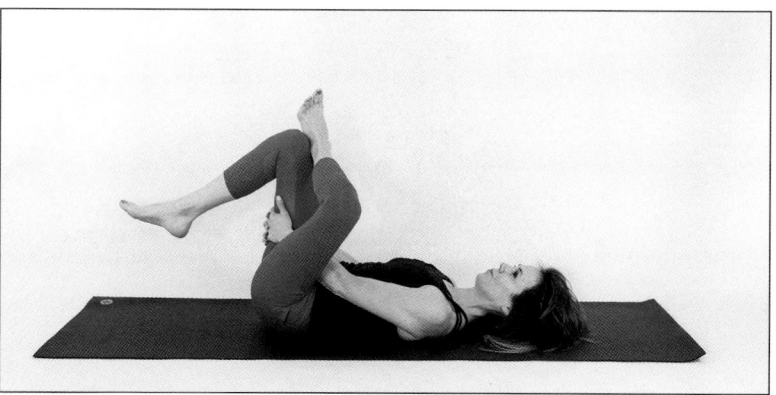

Happy Baby

1. Start lying on your back with your knees bent. Bring your knees toward your armpits. Hold behind your knees, shins, or ankles. Lift your feet toward the ceiling and keep your feet wide apart.
2. Keep the back of your head and upper back in contact with the floor. Gradually move your tailbone closer to the floor.

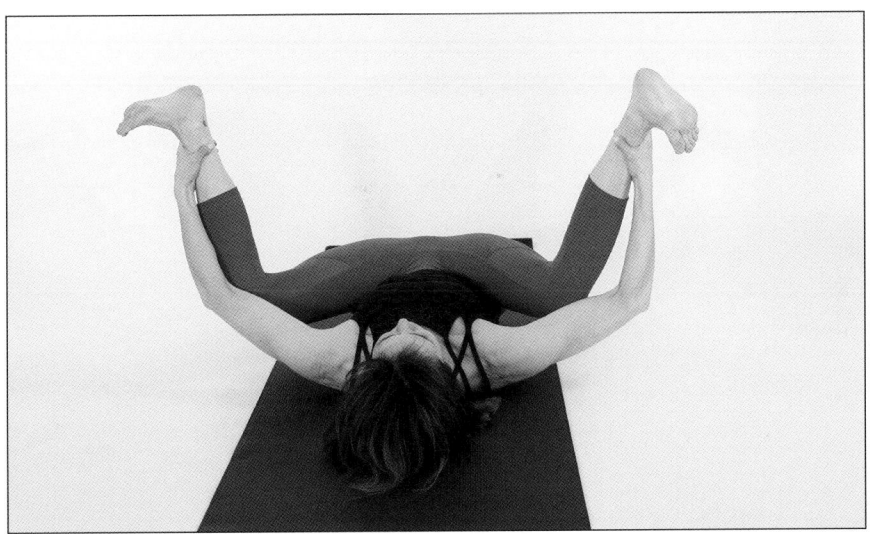

Simple Cross-Legged Seat

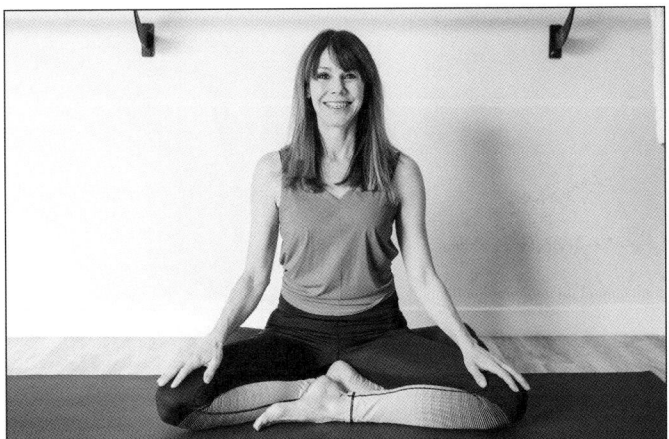

Appendix A

Figure A–1.
The Multidimensional Assessment of Interoceptive Awareness (MAIA) (page 1 of 4)

Multidimensional Assessment of Interoceptive Awareness (Version 2)

Permission and Copyright

Although the MAIA survey is copyrighted, it is available without charge and no written permission is required for its use. This assumes agreement with the following as a consequence of using a MAIA survey:

● Please refer to the survey using its complete name – Multidimensional Assessment of Interoceptive Awareness - and provide the appropriate citation.

● Modifications may be made without our written permission. However, please clearly identify any modifications in any publications as having been made by the users. If you modify the survey, please let us know for our records.

● We recommend including entire subscales when selecting items from the MAIA to retain the psychometric features of these subscales (rather than selecting items from subscales).

● If you translate the MAIA into another language, please send us a copy for our records.

● If other investigators are interested in obtaining the survey, please refer them to the source document (PLoS-ONE 2012, and www.osher.ucsf.edu/maia/) to assure they obtain the most recent version and scoring instructions.

Scoring Instructions

Take the average of the items on each scale.

Note: (R): reverse-score (5 – x) items 5, 6, 7, 8, 9 and 10 on Not-Distracting, and items 11, 12 and 15 on Not-Worrying.

1.   **Noticing:** Awareness of uncomfortable, comfortable, and neutral body sensations

Q1_____ + Q2_____ + Q3_____ + Q4_____ / 4 = _____

2.   **Not-Distracting:** Tendency not to ignore or distract oneself from sensations of pain or discomfort

Q5(**R**)____ + Q6(**R**)____+ Q7(**R**)____+ Q8(**R**)____+Q9(**R**)____+Q10(**R**) / 6 = _____

3.   **Not-Worrying:** Tendency not to worry or experience emotional distress with sensations of pain or discomfort

Q11(**R**)_____ + Q12(**R**)_____ + Q13_____ + Q14_____ + Q15 (**R**) / 5 = _____

4.   **Attention Regulation:** Ability to sustain and control attention to body sensations

Q16_____ + Q17_____ + Q18_____ + Q19_____ + Q20_____ + Q21_____ + Q22_____ / 7 = _____

5.   **Emotional Awareness:** Awareness of the connection between body sensations and emotional states

Q23_____ + Q24_____ + Q25_____ + Q26_____ + Q27_____ / 5 = _____

6.   **Self-Regulation:** Ability to regulate distress by attention to body sensations

Q28_____ + Q29_____ + Q30_____ + Q31_____ / 4= _____

7.   **Body Listening:** Active listening to the body for insight

Q32_____ + Q33_____ + Q34_____ / 3= _____

8.   **Trusting:** Experience of one's body as safe and trustworthy

Q35_____ + Q36_____ + Q37_____ / 3= _____

Figure A–1. (continued)
The Multidimensional Assessment of Interoceptive Awareness (MAIA) (page 2 of 4)

Below you will find a list of statements. Please indicate how often each statement applies to you generally in daily life.

	Circle one number on each line.					
	Never					Always
1. When I am tense I notice where the tension is located in my body.	0	1	2	3	4	5
2. I notice when I am uncomfortable in my body.	0	1	2	3	4	5
3. I notice where in my body I am comfortable.	0	1	2	3	4	5
4. I notice changes in my breathing, such as whether it slows down or speeds up.	0	1	2	3	4	5
5. I ignore physical tension or discomfort until they become more severe.	0	1	2	3	4	5
6. I distract myself from sensations of discomfort.	0	1	2	3	4	5
7. When I feel pain or discomfort, I try to power through it.	0	1	2	3	4	5
8. I try to ignore pain.	0	1	2	3	4	5
9. I push feelings of discomfort away by focusing on something.	0	1	2	3	4	5
10. When I feel unpleasant body sensations, I occupy myself with something else so I don't have to feel them.	0	1	2	3	4	5
11. When I feel physical pain, I become upset.	0	1	2	3	4	5
12. I start to worry that something is wrong if I feel any discomfort.	0	1	2	3	4	5
13. I can notice an unpleasant body sensation without worrying about it.	0	1	2	3	4	5
14. I can stay calm and not worry when I have feelings of discomfort or pain.	0	1	2	3	4	5
15. When I am in discomfort or pain I can't get it out of my mind.	0	1	2	3	4	5
16. I can pay attention to my breath without being distracted by things happening around me.	0	1	2	3	4	5
17. I can maintain awareness of my inner bodily sensations even when there is a lot going on around me.	0	1	2	3	4	5
18. When I am in conversation with someone, I can pay attention to my posture.	0	1	2	3	4	5

Figure A–1. (continued)
The Multidimensional Assessment of Interoceptive Awareness (MAIA) (page 3 of 4)

How often does each statement apply to you generally in daily <u>life? Circle one number on each line.</u>

	Never				Always	
19. I can return awareness to my body if I am distracted.	0	1	2	3	4	5
20. I can refocus my attention from thinking to sensing my body.	0	1	2	3	4	5
21. I can maintain awareness of my whole body even when a part of me is in pain or discomfort.	0	1	2	3	4	5
22. I am able to consciously focus on my body as a whole.	0	1	2	3	4	5
23. I notice how my body changes when I am angry.	0	1	2	3	4	5
24. When something is wrong in my life I can feel it in my body.	0	1	2	3	4	5
25. I notice that my body feels different after a peaceful experience.	0	1	2	3	4	5
26. I notice that my breathing becomes free and easy when I feel comfortable.	0	1	2	3	4	5
27. I notice how my body changes when I feel happy/joyful.	0	1	2	3	4	5
28. When I feel overwhelmed I can find a calm place inside.	0	1	2	3	4	5
29. When I bring awareness to my body I feel a sense of calm.	0	1	2	3	4	5
30. I can use my breath to reduce tension.	0	1	2	3	4	5
31. When I am caught up in thoughts, I can calm my mind by focusing on my body/breathing.	0	1	2	3	4	5
32. I listen for information from my body about my emotional state.	0	1	2	3	4	5
33. When I am upset, I take time to explore how my body feels.	0	1	2	3	4	5
34. I listen to my body to inform me about what to do.	0	1	2	3	4	5
35. I am at home in my body.	0	1	2	3	4	5
36. I feel my body is a safe place.	0	1	2	3	4	5
37. I trust my body sensations.	0	1	2	3	4	5

Figure A–1. (continued)
The Multidimensional Assessment of Interoceptive Awareness (MAIA) (page 4 of 4)

Appendix B

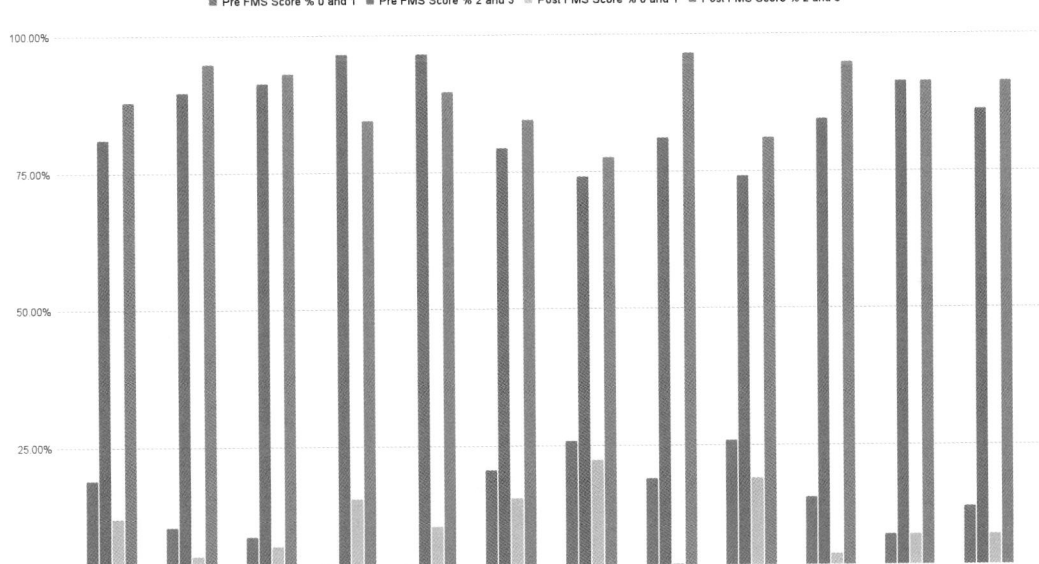

Figure B-1.
Percentage scoring 0 or 1 vs 2 or 3 on each movement pattern on Functional Movement Screen (FMS)

The Functional Movement Screen (FMS) assesses 7 unique movement patterns: Deep Squat, Hurdle Step, Inline Lunge, Shoulder Mobility, Active Straight Leg Raise, Trunk Stability, and Rotary Stability (for more information on the FMS, see their website at https://www. functionalmovement.com/home/sitepage?title=About). Each of the 7 movement patterns in the FMS is given a score between 0 and 3. A score of 0 indicates pain during the movement; a score of 1 indicates a significant amount of overcompensation needed to complete the movement pattern or an inability to complete the movement pattern; a score of 2 indicates a normal and acceptable level of compensation needed to complete the movement pattern; and a score of 3 indicates that the person performed the movement pattern perfectly with no compensation needed.

We compared the number of firefighters who scored a 0 or 1 (indicative of lower than ideal movement function) to the number of firefighters who received a score of 2 or 3 (indicative of acceptable movement function) before and after their 10 session yoga intervention with FireFlex Yoga. We found that in Deep Squat, Hurdle Step, Shoulder Mobility, Active Straight Leg Raise, Trunk Stability, and Rotary Stability (6 of the 7 movement patterns), there was a decrease in scores of 0 or 1 and an increase in scores of 2 or 3.

The only movement pattern to show an increase in scores of 0 or 1 and a decrease in scores of 2 or 3 was the Inline Lunge. This is not surprising, since our 10 session yoga program focuses on mobility and joint stability in the simpler movement patterns first, so that there is a solid foundation from which to build off of. It may be the case that the Inline Lunge would show a similar improvement in those programs that we continued to teach yoga (sessions 11-20), but at this point, we only have data following the initial 10 session yoga program. Further research is needed to discern what trends there may be present in future yoga sessions as firefighters continue their yoga practice past the initial 10 sessions.

In contrast to the FMS, the MAIA scoring system is not designed to derive "hard lines" in terms of functional vs. nonfunctional scores. However, comparisons can be made to regular populations to derive a meaningful "line" between a "normal" score and "abnormal." To find this cutoff line, we used mean data from a study of the general population of museum goers. (See The Multidimensional Assessment of Interoceptive Awareness, Version 2, https://doi.org/10.1371/journal.pone.0208034.t003. It shows the basic descriptive statistics for the eight MAIA scales with Cronbach alphas—scale means and range of item-scale correlations.)

All firefighter scores that fell below one standard deviation of the mean were considered "lower range" scores, while all scores that fell above one standard deviation of the mean were considered "higher range" scores. A large majority of the firefighter population scored *within* this range, which would be considered in this case, "normal range." What is more interesting to note though, is the change from before Fireflex Yoga to after in terms of the percentage of firefighters who initially scored "lower range" vs. "higher range." For example, in the category Noticing, 13.8% scored in the lower range prior to attending FireFlex Yoga. That number dropped to 0 following FireFlex Yoga. What this change means is that there were no firefighters who scored in the "lower range" in the Noticing category after FireFlex Yoga. In this same category, 10.3% of Firefighters scored in the higher range before FireFlex Yoga, and that number increased to 20.7% after FireFlex Yoga.

As can be seen in Figure B-2, there was a general trend of more "higher range" scores on individual scores, and especially noticeable was the change in total score before and after.

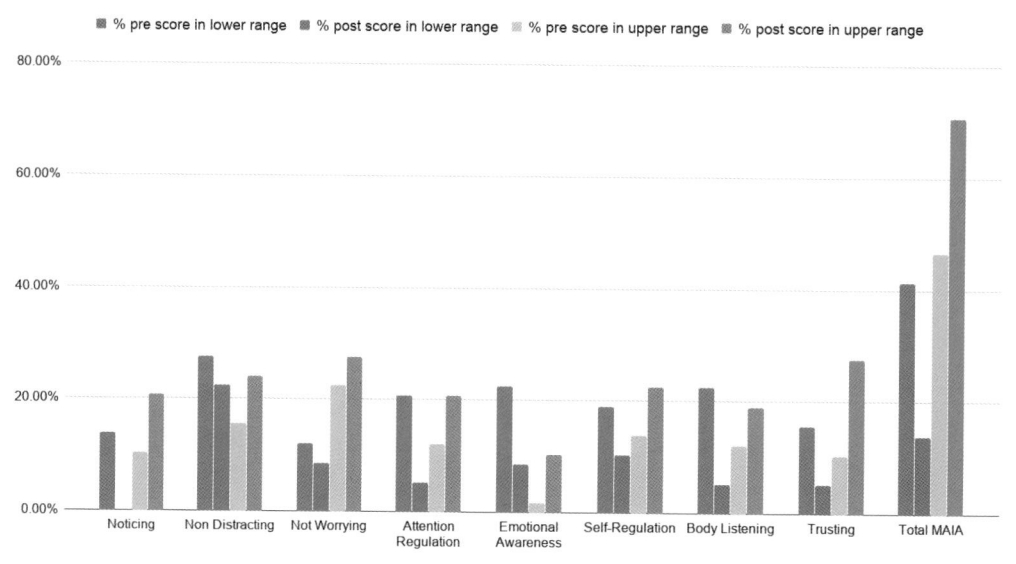

Figure B–2.
Comparing pre and post MAIA scores for firefighters to regular population

Notes

Chapter 1

1   Callahan, Mary, and Christi Warren. 2017. Tubbs Fire in Santa Rosa now ranks as California's most destructive wildfire. *The Press Democrat*. October 20. https://www.pressdemocrat.com/news/7546956-181/tubbs-fire-in-santa-rosa.

2   Ritt, Glenn. n.d. Dealing with Life and Death Daily. Cape and Islands EMS System website. https://www.capeandislandsems.org/4560-2.

3   These two articles give more information on EMS calls: Keisling, Phil. 2015. Why we need to take the "fire" out of "fire department." *Governing: The Future of States and Localities*. June 26. https://www.governing.com/columns/smart-mgmt/col-fire-departments-rethink-delivery-emergency-medical-services.html; Eng, Monica. 2017. Why send a firetruck to do an ambulance's job. NPR. April 11. https://www.npr.org/sections/health-shots/2017/04/11/523025987/why-send-a-firetruck-to-do-an-ambulances-job.

4   Centers for Disease Control and Prevention. n.d. Understanding the epidemic. https://www.cdc.gov/drugoverdose/epidemic/index.html.

5   Coates, Crawford. 2019. *Mindful Responder: The First Responder's Field Guide to Improved Resilience, Fulfillment, Presence, and Fitness—On and Off the Job*. Northbrook, IL: Calibre Press.

6   Marlantes, Karl. 2011. *What It Is Like to Go to War*. New York: Atlantic Monthly Press.

7   Ibid., p. 82.

8   Young-Eisendrath, Polly, and Terence Dawson, eds. 2008. *The Cambridge Companion to Jung*. Cambridge: Cambridge University Press. P. 109. https://www.cambridge.org/core/books/cambridge-companion-to-jung/DCC16E7952C1749A08BAC3F5C7181EC6.

9   Warren, Christy. 2020. Lisa Houle—defense attorney for first responders. The Firefighter Deconstructed podcast. September 29. https://www.spreaker.com/user/mhnrnetwork/lisa-houle-defense-attorney-for-first-re.

10 McCoppin, Robert, Angie Leventis Lourgos, and Alicia Fabbre. 2018. Female fire-fighters still fight for equality: "We're assumed incompetent." *Chicago Tribune*. April 25. Reprinted in: https://www.govtech.com/em/disaster/Female-Firefighter-Still-Fight-for-Equality-Were-assumed-Incompetent.html.

11 Jahnke, Sara. 2019. Fire service stress: Firefighters reflect on the impact of the job. *FireRescue1*. June 17. https://www.firerescue1.com/stress/articles/394330018-Fire-service-stress-Firefighters-reflect-on-the-impact-of-the-job.

12 Marlantes, p. 155.

13 Campbell, Richard, Ben Evarts, and Joseph L. Molis. 2019. *United States Firefighter Injury Report 2018*. National Fire Protection Association.

14 Butry, David T., David Webb, and Stanley Gilbert. 2019. The economics of firefighter injuries in the United States: Executive summary. National Fire Protection Association. Fire Protection Research Foundation. https://www.nfpa.org//-/media/Files/News-and-Research/Fire-statistics-and-reports/Emergency-responders/RFFFCostOfInjuryExecutiveSummary.pdf.

15 Firefighter Cancer Support Network. Firefighter cancer fact check. FirefighterCancerSupport.org. https://www.firefighterclosecalls.com/wp-content/uploads/2017/06/FF-Cancer-Fact-Sheet.pdf.

16 Penn Medicine. 2019. Firefighters and heart health. Penn Heart and Vascular Blog. January 30. https://www.pennmedicine.org/updates/blogs/heart-and-vascular-blog/2019/january/firefighters-and-heart-health.

17 Gill, Rosalynn, Harold Robert Superko, Megan M. McCarthy, Kepra Jack, Briana Jones, Debanjali Ghosh, Steve Richards, Joi A. Gleason, Paul T. Williams, and Michael Dansinger. 2019. Cardiovascular risk factor reduction in first responders resulting from an individualized lifestyle and blood test program. *Journal of Occupational and Environmental Medicine*. 61 (3): 183–189. https://www.ncbi.nlm.nih.gov/pmc/articles/PMC6416033/.

18 Substance Abuse and Mental Health Services Administration. 2018. First responders: Behavioral health concerns, emergency response, and trauma. *Disaster Technical Assistance Center Supplemental Research Bulletin*. May. https://www.samhsa.gov/sites/default/files/dtac/supplementalresearchbulletin-firstresponders-may2018.pdf.

19 Ushery, David, Evan Stulberger, Liz Wagner, Michael Bott, and Dave Manney. 2018. I-Team: National data shows firefighters' mental, emotional health not getting enough attention. NBC New York. February 22, updated March 19. https://www.nbcnewyork.com/news/local/Firefighters-Mental-Health-Survey-PTSD-474859323.html.

Chapter 2

1 Pressfield, Steven. n.d. The war inside ourselves. Steven Pressfield blog. https://stevenpressfield.com/2011/04/the-war-inside-ourselves.

2 Mayo Clinic Staff. 2020. Yoga: Fight stress and find serenity. Mayo Clinic website. December 29. https://www.mayoclinic.org/healthy-lifestyle/stress-management/in-depth/yoga/art-20044733.

3 Harvard Health Publishing. 2020. Increased well-being: Another reason to try yoga. August 24. https://www.health.harvard.edu/mind-and-mood/increased-well-being-another-reason-to-try-yoga.

4 American Osteopathic Association. n.d. The benefits of yoga. https://osteopathic.org/what-is-osteopathic-medicine/benefits-of-yoga.

5 United States Army Inspector General Agency. 2010. *Inspection of the Warrior Care and Transition Program*. http://graphics8.nytimes.com/packages/pdf/us/10drugs-WCTP-Insp-Rpt1.pdf.

6 Drug Policy Alliance. 2012. Healing a broken system: Veterans and the war on drugs. November. https://www.drugpolicy.org/sites/default/files/DPA_Healing%20a%20Broken%20System_Veterans%20and%20the%20War%20on%20Drugs_November%202012_Final_0.pdf.

7   National Institute on Drug Abuse. 2019. Substance use and military life. Drug Facts. October. https://www.drugabuse.gov/publications/drugfacts/substance-use-military-life.

8   Highland, Krista Beth, Audrey Schoomaker, Winifred Rojas, Josh Suen, Ambareen Ahmed, Zhiwei Zhang, Sarah Fink Carlin, et al. 2018. Benefits of the restorative exercise and strength training for operational resilience and excellence yoga program for chronic low back pain in service members: A pilot randomized controlled trial. *Physical Medicine and Rehabilitation*. 99 (1): 91–98. https://www.ncbi.nlm.nih.gov/pubmed/28919191/.

9   Tucker, Lindsay. 2018. The good fight: How yoga is being used within the military. *Yoga Journal*. September 27. https://www.yogajournal.com/lifestyle/how-yoga-is-being-used-within-the-military.

Chapter 3

1   Brezler, Jason. 2017. Mental toughness on the battlefield and the fireground with FDNY firefighter and US Marine Corps Major Jason Brezler. FDNY Pro podcast. S2, E14. http://www.fdnypro.org/podcast/one-on-one-with-firefighter-and-us-marine-corps-major-jason-brezler/.

2   Mullen, M. G. 2011. *Chairman of the Joint Chiefs of Staff Instruction*. Enclosure A—Chairman's total force fitness framework. Appendix F—Psychological fitness. September 1. https://www.jcs.mil/Portals/36/Documents/Library/Instructions/3405_01.pdf.

3   Substance Abuse and Mental Health Services Administration. 2018. First responders: Behavioral health concerns, emergency response, and trauma. *Disaster Technical Assistance Center Supplemental Research Bulletin*. May. https://www.samhsa.gov/sites/default/files/dtac/supplementalresearchbulletin-firstresponders-may2018.pdf.

4   Hardasmalani, Madhu. 2017. Bouncing back: Building resilience through yoga. *Emergency Medicine News*. 39 (8): 35, 37. https://journals.lww.com/em-news/FullText/2017/08000/Bouncing_Back__Building_Resilience_through_Yoga.20.aspx.

5   Davidson, Richard. "From states to traits: The latest science on what meditation can and can't do.," Interview by Marianne Spoon. University of Wisconsin–Madison Center for Healthy Minds. 2021. https://centerhealthyminds.org/join-the-movement/from-states-to-traits-uws-richard-davidson-shares-latest-science-on-what-meditation-can-and-cant-do.

6   Mindful Staff. 2020. What is mindfulness? *Mindful*. July 8. https://www.mindful.org/what-is-mindfulness/.

7   Mindful Staff. 2017. Jon Kabat-Zinn: Defining mindfulness. *Mindful*. January 11. https://www.mindful.org/jon-kabat-zinn-defining-mindfulness/.

8   Mindfulness Program, University of Arkansas for Medical Science. n.d. Mindfulness. https://mindfulness.uams.edu/science/.

9   Williamson, Mark, and Renata Salecl. n.d. Autopilot Britain. https://corporate.marksandspencer.com/documents/reports-results-and-publications/autopilot-britain-whitepaper.pdf.

10 Khalsa, Sahib S., Ralph Adolphs, Oliver G. Cameron, Hugo D. Critchley, Paul W. Davenport, Justin S. Feinstein, Jamie D. Feusner, et al. 2018. Interoception and mental health: A roadmap. *Biological Psychiatry*: *Cognitive Neuroscience and*

Neuroimaging. 3 (6): 501–513. https://www.ncbi.nlm.nih.gov/pmc/articles/PMC6054486/.

11 Worrall, Simon. 2018. Why the brain-body connection is more important than we think. *National Geographic.* March 17. https://www.nationalgeographic.com/news/2018/03/why-the-brain-body-connection-is-more-important-than-we-think.

12 Maull, Fleet. 2020. An introduction to neuro-somatic mindfulness. Heart Mind Institute podcast. October 27. https://hmi.fleetmaull.com/FSb251.

13 Farb, Norman, and Wolf E. Mehling. 2016. Interoception, contemplative practice, and health. *Frontiers in Psychology.* December 1. https://www.frontiersin.org/articles/10.3389/fpsyg.2016.01898/full.

14 St. Michael's Hospital. n.d. Mindfulness and the window of tolerance. Mindful Awareness Stabilization Training (M.A.S.T.). Session 1. http://www.rachaelfrankford.com/uploads/6/9/4/5/69457525/mast_session_1.pdf.

15 Barrett, Lisa Feldman, and W. Kyle Simmons. 2015. Interoceptive predictions in the brain. *Nature Reviews Neuroscience.* 16: 419–429. https://www.nature.com/articles/nrn3950.

16 Craig, A. D. 2011. A. D. (Bud) Craig on the anterior insula and human awareness. ScienceWatch.com. May. http://archive.sciencewatch.com/dr/fmf/2011/11mayfmf/11mayfmfCrai/.

17 Chen, Wen G., Dana Schloesser, Angela M. Arensdorf, Janine M. Simmons, Changhai Cui, Rita Valentino, James W. Gnadt, et al. 2021. The emerging science of interoception: Sensing, integrating, interpreting, and regulating signals within the self. *Trends in Neuroscience.* 44 (1): 3–16. https://doi.org/10.1016/j.tins.2020.10.007.

18 Haase, Lori, Nate J. Thom, Akanksha Shukla, Paul W. Davenport, Alan N. Simmons, Elizabeth A. Stanley, Martin P. Paulus, and Douglas C. Johnson. 2014. Mindfulness-based training attenuates insula response to an aversive interoceptive challenge. *Social Cognitive and Affective Neuroscience.* 11 (1): 182–190. https://www.ncbi.nlm.nih.gov/pmc/articles/PMC4692309/.

19 Dweck, Carol. 2007. *Mindset: The New Psychology of Success.* Updated ed. New York: Ballantine Books.

Chapter 4

1 Scott, Elizabeth. 2019. When stress is actually good for you. The American Institute of Stress website. November 18. https://www.stress.org/when-stress-is-actually-good-for-you.

2 St. Michael's Hospital. n.d. Mindfulness and the window of tolerance. Mindful Awareness Stabilization Training (M.A.S.T.). Session 1. http://www.rachaelfrankford.com/uploads/6/9/4/5/69457525/mast_session_1.pdf.

3 Harvard Health Publishing. 2018. Understanding the stress response. May 1. https://www.health.harvard.edu/staying-healthy/understanding-the-stress-response.

4 Kotas, Maya E., and Ruslan Medzhitov. 2015. Homeostasis, inflammation, and disease susceptibility. *Cell.* 160 (5): 816–827. https://www.cell.com/fulltext/S0092-8674(15)00175-0.

5 Carnegie Mellon University. 2012. How stress influences disease: Study reveals inflammation as the culprit. *ScienceDaily.* April 2. https://www.sciencedaily.com/releases/2012/04/120402162546.htm.

6   Mayo Clinic Staff. 2019. Chronic stress puts your health at risk. Mayo Clinic website. March 19. https://www.mayoclinic.org/healthy-lifestyle/stress-management/in-depth/stress/art-20046037.

7   Herman, James P., Jessica M. McKlveen, Sriparna Ghosal, Brittany Kopp, Aynara Wulsin, Ryan Makinson, Jessie Scheimann, and Brent Myers. 2016. Regulation of the hypothalamic-pituitary-adrenocortical stress response. *Comprehensive Physiology.* 6 (2): 603–621. https://www.ncbi.nlm.nih.gov/pmc/articles/PMC4867107/.

8   Stephens, Mary Ann C., and Gary Wand. 2012. Stress and the HPA axis: Role of glucocorticoids in alcohol dependence. *Alcohol Research: Current Reviews.* 34 (4): 468–483. https://www.ncbi.nlm.nih.gov/pmc/articles/PMC3860380/.

9   Smith, Joshua P., and Carrie L. Randall. 2012. Anxiety and alcohol use disorders: Comorbidity and treatment considerations. *Alcohol Research: Current Reviews.* 34 (4): 414–431. https://www.ncbi.nlm.nih.gov/pubmed/23584108/.

10 Behar, Michael. 2014. Can the nervous system be hacked? *New York Times Magazine.* May 23. https://www.nytimes.com/2014/05/25/magazine/can-the-nervous-system-be-hacked.html.

11 Goldman, Bruce. 2017. Study shows how slow breathing induces tranquility. Stanford Medicine News Center. March 30. https://med.stanford.edu/news/all-news/2017/03/study-discovers-how-slow-breathing-induces-tranquility.html.

Chapter 5

1   Merz, C. Noel Bairey, Omeed Elboudwarej, and Puja Mehta. 2015. The autonomic nervous system and cardiovascular health and disease: A complex balancing act. *JACC: Heart Failure.* 3 (5): 383–385. http://heartfailure.onlinejacc.org/content/3/5/383.

2   de Vente, Wieke, Jan G. C. van Amsterdam, Miranda Olff, Jan H. Kamphuis, and Paul M. G. Emmelkamp. 2015. Burnout is associated with reduced parasympathetic activity and reduced HPA axis responsiveness, predominantly in males. *BioMed Research International.* 2015: 431725. https://www.ncbi.nlm.nih.gov/pmc/articles/PMC4628754/.

3   Fioranelli, Massimo, Anna G. Bottaccioli, Francesco Bottaccioli, Maria Bianchi, Miriam Rovesti, and Maria G. Roccia. 2018. Stress and inflammation in coronary artery disease: A review psychoneuroendocrineimmunology-based. *Frontiers in Immunology.* September 6. https://www.frontiersin.org/articles/10.3389/fimmu.2018.02031/full.

4   Johns Hopkins Medicine. n.d. The yoga-heart connection. https://www.hopkinsmedicine.org/health/wellness-and-prevention/the-yoga-heart-connection.

5   Pascoe, Michaela C., David R. Thompson, Zoe M. Jenkins, and Chantal F. Ski. 2017. Mindfulness mediates the physiological markers of stress: Systematic review and meta-analysis. *Journal of Psychiatric Research.* 95 (December): 156–178. https://www.sciencedirect.com/science/article/abs/pii/S0022395617301462.

6   Campos, Marcelo. 2019. Heart rate variability: A new way to track well-being. Harvard Health Publishing. October 22. https://www.health.harvard.edu/blog/heart-rate-variability-new-way-track-well-2017112212789.

7   Vinay, A. V., D. Venkatesh, and V. Ambarish. 2016. Impact of short-term practice of yoga on heart rate variability. *International Journal of Yoga.* 9 (1): 62–66. https://www.ncbi.nlm.nih.gov/pmc/articles/PMC4728961/.

8   Jouvenal, Justin. 2019. New survey shows heavy psychological toll for Virginia's first responders. *Washington Post.* September 10. https://www.washingtonpost.com/local/

public-safety/new-survey-shows-heavy-psychological-toll-for-vas-first-responders/
2019/09/09/636df99e-d323-11e9-9610-fb56c5522e1c_story.html.

9   Yang, Longfei, Yinghao Zhao, Yicun Wang, Lei Liu, Xingyi Zhang, Bingjin Li, and
    Ranji Cuia. 2015. The effects of psychological stress on depression. *Current
    Neuropharmacology*. 13 (4): 494–504. https://www.ncbi.nlm.nih.gov/pmc/articles/
    PMC4790405/.

10 Miller, Andrew H., Ebrahim Haroon, Charles L. Raison, and Jennifer C. Felger. 2013.
    Cytokine targets in the brain: Impact on neurotransmitters and neurocircuits.
    Depression and Anxiety. 30 (4): 297–306. https://www.ncbi.nlm.nih.gov/pmc/articles/
    PMC4141874/.

11 N. Vogelzangs, P. de Jonge, J. H. Smit, S. Bahn, and B. W. Penninx. 2016. Cytokine
    production capacity in depression and anxiety. *Translational Psychiatry*. 6 (5): e825.
    https://www.ncbi.nlm.nih.gov/pmc/articles/PMC5070051/; Raison, Charles L., Lucile
    Capuron, and Andrew H. Miller. 2006. Cytokines sing the blues: Inflammation and
    the pathogenesis of depression. *Trends in Immunology*. 27 (1): 24–31. https://www.
    ncbi.nlm.nih.gov/pmc/articles/PMC3392963/.

12 Ganança, Licínia, Maria A. Oquendo, Audrey R. Tyrka, Sebastian Cisneros-Trujillo, J.
    John Mann, and M. Elizabeth Sublette. 2016. The role of cytokines in the pathophys-
    iology of suicidal behavior," *Psychoneuroendocrinology*, 63 (January): 296–310. https://
    www.ncbi.nlm.nih.gov/pmc/articles/PMC4910882/.

13 Breit, Sigrid, Aleksandra Kupferberg, Gerhard Rogler, and Gregor Hasler. 2018. Vagus
    nerve as modulator of the brain-gut axis in psychiatric and inflammatory disorders.
    Frontiers in Psychiatry. 9: 44. https://www.ncbi.nlm.nih.gov/pmc/articles/
    PMC5859128/.

14 Wei, Marlynn. 2020. Yoga could slow the harmful effects of stress and inflamma-
    tion. Harvard Health Publishing. August 10. https://www.health.harvard.edu/blog/
    yoga-could-slow-the-harmful-effects-of-stress-and-inflammation-2017101912588.

15 Sonnenburg, Justin, and Erica Sonnenburg. 2015. Gut feelings—the "second brain"
    in our gastrointestinal systems [excerpt]. *Scientific American*. May 1. https://www.
    scientificamerican.com/article/gut-feelings-the-second-brain-in-our-gastrointestinal-
    systems-excerpt.

16 Klarer, Melanie, Myrtha Arnold, Lydia Günther, Christine Winter, Wolfgang
    Langhans, and Urs Meyer. 2014. Gut vagal afferents differentially modulate innate
    anxiety and learned fear. *Journal of Neuroscience*. 34 (21): 7067–7076. https://www.
    jneurosci.org/content/34/21/7067.

17 Stephenson, Kyle R., Tracy L. Simpson, Michelle E. Martinez, and David J. Kearney.
    2017. Changes in mindfulness and posttraumatic stress disorder symptoms among
    veterans enrolled in mindfulness-based stress reduction. *Journal of Clinical Psychology*.
    73 (3): 201–217. https://pubmed.ncbi.nlm.nih.gov/27152480/.

18 Stanley, Ian H., Joseph W. Boffa, Jana K. Tran, Norman Brad Schmidt, Thomas E.
    Joiner, and Anka A. Vujanovic. 2019. Posttraumatic stress disorder symptoms and
    mindfulness facets in relation to suicide risk among firefighters. *Journal of Clinical
    Psychology*. 75 (4): 696–709. https://www.ncbi.nlm.nih.gov/pmc/articles/
    PMC6434694/.

19 Alexander, Walter. 2012. Pharmacotherapy for post-traumatic stress disorder in
    combat veterans: Focus on antidepressants and atypical antipsychotic agents.
    Pharmacy and Therapeutics. 37 (1): 32–38. https://www.ncbi.nlm.nih.gov/pmc/
    articles/PMC3278188/.

20 Bieman, Jennifer. 2019. Study of yoga treatment for PTSD clinches federal funding. *London Free Press*. February 8. https://lfpress.com/news/local-news/study-of-yoga-treatment-for-ptsd-clinches-federal-funding.

21 Brigham and Women's Hospital. 2014. Sleep disorders found to be highly prevalent in firefighters. *ScienceDaily*. November 13. https://www.sciencedaily.com/releases/2014/11/141113085220.htm.

22 Harvard Health Publishing. 2019. Sleep and mental health. March 18. https://www.health.harvard.edu/newsletter_article/sleep-and-mental-health.

23 Tobaldini, Eleonora, Giorgio Costantino, Monica Solbiati, Chiara Cogliati, Tomas Kara, Lino Nobili, and Nicola Montano. 2017. Sleep, sleep deprivation, autonomic nervous system and cardiovascular diseases. *Neuroscience and Biobehavioral Review*. 74 (part B): 321–329. https://www.sciencedirect.com/science/article/abs/pii/S0149763416302184.

24 Fioranelli et al. 2018.

25 Black, David S., Gillian A. O'Reilly, Richard Olmstead, Elizabeth C. Breen, and Michael R. Irwin. 2015. Mindfulness meditation and improvement in sleep quality and daytime impairment among older adults with sleep disturbances: A randomized clinical trial. *JAMA Internal Medicine*. 175 (4): 494–501. https://jamanetwork.com/journals/jamainternalmedicine/fullarticle/2110998.

26 Ong, Jason C., Rachel Manber, Zindel Segal, Yinglin Xia, Shauna Shapiro, and James K. Wyatt. 2014. A randomized controlled trial of mindfulness meditation for chronic insomnia. *Sleep*. 37 (9): 1553–1563. https://www.ncbi.nlm.nih.gov/pmc/articles/PMC4153063/.

27 Zhang, Yin, and Kyriaki Papantoniou. 2019. Night shift work and its carcinogenicity. *Lancet Oncology*. 20 (10): e550. https://www.thelancet.com/journals/lanonc/article/PIIS1470-2045(19)30578-9/fulltext.

28 Bullen Love, Danielle. 2017. Circadian rhythm disruption and the link to cancer risk. *Oncology Times*. 39 (16): 1, 5. https://journals.lww.com/oncology-times/fulltext/2017/08250/circadian_rhythm_disruption___the_link_to_cancer.2.aspx.

29 Vinther, Anna Gry, and Mogens H. Claesson. 2015. The influence of melatonin on immune system and cancer. *International Journal of Cancer and Clinical Research*. 2: 4. https://clinmedjournals.org/articles/ijccr/international-journal-of-cancer-and-clinical-research-ijccr-2-024.pdf.

30 Bernstein, Lenny. 2019. For some with chronic pain, the problem is not in their backs or knees but their brains. *Washington Post*. September 23. https://www.washingtonpost.com/national/health-science/for-some-with-chronic-pain-the-problem-is-not-in-their-backs-or-knees-but-their-brains/2019/09/23/80538660-5d5c-11e9-842d-7d3ed7eb3957_story.html.

31 Hannibal, Kara E., and Mark D. Bishop. 2014. Chronic stress, cortisol dysfunction, and pain: A psychoneuroendocrine rationale for stress management in pain rehabilitation. *Physical Therapy*. 94 (12): 1816–1825. https://www.ncbi.nlm.nih.gov/pmc/articles/PMC4263906/.

32 Ibid.

33 Gard, Tim, Jessica J. Noggle, Crystal L. Park, David R. Vago, and Angela Wilson. 2014. Potential self-regulatory mechanisms of yoga for psychological health. *Frontiers in Human Neuroscience*. 8: 770. https://www.ncbi.nlm.nih.gov/pmc/articles/PMC4179745/.

Chapter 6

1   Cook, Gray. 2015. Movement principles. FMS website. December 10. https://www. functionalmovement.com/articles/655/movement_principles.

2   Frost, David M., Tyson A. C. Beach, Jack P. Callaghan, and Stuart M. McGill. 2012. Using the Functional Movement Screen™ to evaluate the effectiveness of training. *Journal of Strength and Conditioning Research*. 26 (6): 1620–1630. https://journals.lww. com/nsca-jscr/Fulltext/2012/06000/Using_the_Functional_Movement_Screen__to_ Evaluate.23.aspx.

3   Phillips, Noelle. 2016. How the Denver Fire Department is treating firefighters like pro athletes to get them back to work. *Denver Post*. December 28. https://www. denverpost.com/2016/12/28/denver-fire-department-rehab; Burton, Lee. 2020. FMS in business: Denver Fire Department. FMS podcast. January 24. https://www. functionalmovement.com/articles/897/fms_in_business_denver_fire_department.

4   Stranek, Justin M., Daniel J. Dodd, Adam R. Kelly, Alex M. Wolfe, and Ryan A. Swenson. 2017. Active duty firefighters can improve Functional Movement Screen (FMS) scores following an 8-week individualized client workout program. *Work*. 56 (2): 213–220. https://content.iospress.com/articles/work/wor2493.

5   Wells, Greg. 1998. Peak performance: A literature review. ResearchGate. December. https://www.researchgate.net/publication/265616014_Peak_Performance_A_ Literature_Review.

6   Mehling, Wolf. 2020. Conversation with author in May.

7   van der Kolk, Bessel. 2014. *The Body Keeps the Score: Brain, Mind, and Body in the Healing of Trauma*. New York: Viking. Pp. 95–96.

8   Rensel, Mary R., and Carrie M. Hersch. n.d. A brain health guide: Multiple sclerosis (MS). Cleveland Clinic. https://my.clevelandclinic.org/-/scassets/files/org/locations/ nevada/multiple-sclerosis/2020-cclr-brain-guide-ms.ashx.

9   The first of these two articles on neuroplasticity presents an easy-to-understand explanation of motor neurons and strength training, and the second article is a general study of neuroplasticity: Oby, Emily R., Matthew D. Golub, Jay A. Hennig, Alan D. Degenhart, Elizabeth C. Tyler-Kabara, Byron M. Yu, Steven M. Chase, and Aaron P. Batista. 2019. New neural activity patterns emerge with long-term learning. *Proceedings of the National Academy of Sciences*. 116 (30): 15210–15215. https://www. pnas.org/content/116/30/15210; Lee, Min Chul, Kyeongho Byun, Ji-Seok Kim, Hojun Lee, and Kijeong Kim. 2019. Trends in exercise neuroscience: Raising demand for brain fitness. *Journal of Exercise Rehabilitation*. 15 (2): 176–179. https://www.ncbi.nlm. nih.gov/pmc/articles/PMC6509468/.

10 This article features a transcript of a podcast with Rick Hanson, one of the leading writers on the subject of neuroplasticity and the science of happiness: Bergeisen, Michael. 2010. The neuroscience of happiness. *Greater Good Magazine*. September 22. https://greatergood.berkeley.edu/article/item/the_neuroscience_of_happiness; Hanson's website also features fun and easy-to-understand explanations of how change works in the brain: https://www.rickhanson.net/the-science-of-positive-brain-change.

11 This meta-review of 18 studies, with more than 800 participants over 11 years, shows compelling evidence of how yoga, mindfulness, and breathing practices can reverse effects of chronic stress by changing the molecular structure of how certain genes express themselves, thereby positively affecting our physical and mental health: Buric, Ivana, Miguel Farias, Jonathan Jong, Christopher Mee, and Inti A. Brazil. 2017. What is the molecular signature of mind–body interventions? A

systematic review of gene expression changes induced by meditation and related practices." *Frontiers in Immunology.* 8: 670. https://www.ncbi.nlm.nih.gov/pmc/articles/PMC5472657/.

Chapter 9

1   Kibler, W. Ben, Joel Press, and Aaron Sciascia. 2006. The role of core stability in athletic function. *Sports Medicine.* 36 (3): 189–198. https://link.springer.com/article/10.2165/00007256-200636030-00001.
2   Kennedy, Tricia. 2011. How combat breathing saved my life. *Police Magazine.* March 9. https://www.policemag.com/373760/how-combat-breathing-saved-my-life.
3   van der Kolk, Bessel. 2014. *The Body Keeps the Score: Brain, Mind, and Body in the Healing of Trauma.* New York: Viking.

Chapter 10

1   Harvard Health Publishing. 2012. The real-world benefits of strengthening your core. January 24. https://www.health.harvard.edu/healthbeat/the-real-world-benefits-of-strengthening-your-core.
2   Mayo Clinic Staff. 2020. Core exercises: Why you should strengthen your core muscles. Mayo Clinic website. August 29. https://www.mayoclinic.org/healthy-lifestyle/fitness/in-depth/core-exercises/art-20044751.
3   Loehr, Jim, and Tony Schwartz. 2001. The making of a corporate athlete. *Harvard Business Review.* January. https://hbr.org/2001/01/the-making-of-a-corporate-athlete.
4   Schwartz, Tony. 2010. Six ways to supercharge your productivity. *Harvard Business Review.* September 7. https://hbr.org/2010/09/six-ways-to-supercharge-your-p-2.
5   For a more detailed explanation of downward-facing dog and other yoga poses, as well as ujjayi breathing, I highly recommend this book: Stephens, Mark. 2010. *Teaching Yoga: Essential Foundations and Techniques.* Berkeley, CA: North Atlantic Books.

Chapter 11

1   Friese, Greg. 2017. Importance of situational awareness process for firefighters. *FireRescue1.* February 15. https://www.firerescue1.com/situational-awareness/articles/importance-of-situational-awareness-process-for-firefighters-HWUS4JoADKGBqxRx.
2   Jha, Amishi. 2017. How to tame your wandering mind. TEDxCoconutGrove video. March 23. https://www.ted.com/talks/amishi_jha_how_to_tame_your_wandering_mind.
3   Baum, Isadora. 2017. "5 Signs that your glutes are weak as hell. *Men's Health.* December 1. https://www.menshealth.com/fitness/a19544187/5-signs-you-have-weak-glutes.
4   This article gives a clear, nonmedical description of the effects of prolonged sitting. Besides, the title is great! Cleveland Clinic HealthEssentials. 2020. No joke: Your desk job promotes "dead butt" syndrome. Cleveland Clinic. August 28. https://health.clevelandclinic.org/no-joke-your-desk-job-promotes-dead-butt-syndrome/.

5   These two academic studies provide detailed descriptions of the effects of balancing exercises on the brain: Dunsky, Ayelet. 2019. The effect of balance and coordination exercises on quality of life in older adults: A mini-review. *Frontiers in Aging Neuroscience*. November 15. https://www.frontiersin.org/articles/10.3389/fnagi.2019.00318/full; Rogge, Ann-Kathrin, Brigitte Röder, Astrid Zech, Volker Nagel, Karsten Hollander, Klaus-Michael Braumann, and Kirsten Hötting. 2017. Balance training improves memory and spatial cognition in healthy adults. *Scientific Reports*. 7: 5661. https://www.ncbi.nlm.nih.gov/pmc/articles/PMC5515881/.

6   Ghiya, Shreya. 2017. Alternate nostril breathing: A systematic review of clinical trials. *International Journal of Research in Medical Sciences*. August. 5 (8): 3273–3286. https://www.msjonline.org/index.php/ijrms/article/view/3581/3158.

Chapter 12

1   Loehr, Jim, and Tony Schwartz. 2001. The making of a corporate athlete. *Harvard Business Review*. January. https://hbr.org/2001/01/the-making-of-a-corporate-athlete.

2   In this inspiring video, General President Harold Schaitberger talks with IAFF members who have struggled with and recovered from posttraumatic stress: Schaitberger, Harold, and IAFF members. 2016. Kitchen table: Overcoming post-traumatic stress. YouTube video. August 13. https://www.youtube.com/watch?v=qk1Ujbbf6Wk.

3   Carter, C. Sue, and Stephen W. Porges. 2013. Neurobiology and the evolution of mammalian social behavior. In D. Narvaez, J. Panksepp, A. N. Schore, and T. R. Gleason, eds. *Evolution, Early Experience and Human Development: From Research to Practice and Policy*. Oxford: Oxford University Press. 132–151. https://psycnet.apa.org/record/2013-01219-008.

4   Stephen Porges is not only a brilliant scientist, but he is also a great explainer. In this interview, he explains the most complex processes in a way that makes you excited to know more about how the body and emotions really work: Porges, Stephen. 2015. The polyvagal theory and the vagal nerve. Bulletproof Radio. December 1 (no. 264). https://art19.com/shows/bulletproof-radio/episodes/27c8187e-a25b-4c97-968f-6ec497decc60.

5   Even if you hate exercising, this article will get you moving: McGonigal, Kelly. 2020. Here's how exercise reduces anxiety and makes you feel more connected. *Washington Post*. January 21. https://www.washingtonpost.com/lifestyle/2020/01/21/heres-how-exercise-reduces-anxiety-makes-you-feel-more-connected.

6   Kaplan, Joshua Benjamin, Aaron L. Bergman, Michael Christopher, Sarah Bowen, and Matthew Hunsinger. 2017. Role of resilience in mindfulness training for first responders. *Mindfulness*. 8: 1373–1380. https://www.researchgate.net/publication/316251337_Role_of_Resilience_in_Mindfulness_Training_for_First_Responders.

7   Zimmerman, Jamie, and Lana Zak. 2015. The secret weapon of CEOs and basketball pros to get in the zone. ABC News. February 18. https://abcnews.go.com/Health/secret-weapon-ceos-basketball-pros-zone/story?id=29051073.

8   Mascaro, Jennifer S., Alana Darcher, Lobsang T. Negi, and Charles L. Raison. 2015. The neural mediators of kindness-based meditation: a theoretical model. *Frontiers in Psychology*. 6: 109. https://www.ncbi.nlm.nih.gov/pmc/articles/PMC4325657/.

9   American Psychological Association. 2012. Building your resilience. https://www.apa.org/topics/resilience.

Chapter 13

1 Warren, Thomas. 2018. Fire service leadership basics: Roles, responsibilities, and boundaries. *Fire Engineering.* June 14. https://www.fireengineering.com/leadership/fire-service-leadership-basics-roles-responsibilities-and-boundaries/#gref.

2 Lorber, Jo-Ann. 2016. Five core competencies of executive leadership. International Fire Chiefs Association website. August 1. https://www.iafc.org/iCHIEFS/iCHIEFS-article/five-core-competencies-of-executive-leadership.

3 Johnson, Christina. 2014. Mindfulness training program may help Olympic athletes reach peak performance. *thisweek@ucsandiego.* June 5. https://ucsdnews.ucsd.edu/feature/mindfulness_training_program_may_help_olympic_athletes_reach_peak.

4 Warren, Thomas. 2017. Command presence: What is it, and how do you develop it? *Fire Engineering.* February 2. https://www.fireengineering.com/leadership/command-presence-what-is-it-and-how-do-you-develop-it/#gref.

5 Goleman, Daniel, and Richard J. Davidson. 2017. *Altered Traits: Science Reveals How Meditation Changes Your Mind, Brain, and Body.* New York: Avery. Pp. 104–105.

6 Cefalu, Joe. 2020. The growth mindset with Lt. Richard Goerling (ret.) "The Han Solo" of mindfulness. The Mindful Cops podcast. April 25 (no. 7). https://anchor.fm/joe-cefalu/episodes/Episode-007-The-Growth-Mindset-with-Lt--Richard-Goerling-ret--The-Han-Solo-of-Mindfulness-eco2bl.

7 Kearney, David J., Carol A. Malte, Carolyn McManus, Michelle E. Martinez, Ben Felleman, and Tracy L. Simpson. 2013. Loving-kindness meditation for posttraumatic stress disorder: A pilot study. *Journal of Traumatic Stress.* 26 (4): 426–434. https://pubmed.ncbi.nlm.nih.gov/23893519/.

8 Shahar, Ben, Ohad Szsepsenwol, Sigal Zilcha-Mano, Netalee Haim, Orly Zamir, Simi Levi-Yeshuvi, and Nava Levit-Binnun. 2015. A wait-list randomized controlled trial of loving-kindness meditation programme for self-criticism. *Clinical Psychology and Psychotherapy.* 22 (4): 346–356. https://pubmed.ncbi.nlm.nih.gov/24633992/.

9 Hutcherson, Cendri A., Emma M. Seppala, and James J. Gross. 2008. Loving-kindness meditation increases social connectedness. Emotion. 8 (5): 720–724. https://contextualscience.org/system/files/Hutcherson,2008.pdf.

Index